Career Guide
for Nurse Educators

Career Guide for Nurse Educators

Margaret Denise Zanecchia, Ph.D., R.N.
Associate Professor
College of Nursing
Texas Christian University
Fort Worth, Texas

APPLETON & LANGE
Norwalk, Connecticut/San Mateo, California

0-8385-1080-9

Notice: The author(s) and publisher of this volume have taken care that the information and recommendations contained herein are accurate and compatible with the standards generally accepted at the time of publication.

Copyright © 1988 by Appleton & Lange
A Publishing Division of Prentice Hall

All rights reserved. This book, or any parts thereof, may not be used or reproduced in any manner without written permission. For information, address Appleton & Lange, 25 Van Zant Street, East Norwalk, Connecticut 06855.

88 89 90 91 92 / 10 9 8 7 6 5 4 3 2 1

Prentice-Hall of Australia, Pty. Ltd., Sydney
Prentice-Hall Canada, Inc.
Prentice-Hall Hispanoamericana, S.A., Mexico
Prentice-Hall of India Private Limited, New Delhi
Prentice-Hall International (UK) Limited, London
Prentice-Hall of Japan, Inc., Tokyo
Prentice-Hall of Southeast Asia (Pte.) Ltd., Singapore
Whitehall Books Ltd., Wellington, New Zealand
Editora Prentice-Hall do Brasil Ltda., Rio de Janeiro

Library of Congress Cataloging-in-Publication Data

Zanecchia, Margaret Denise.
  Career guide for nurse educators.

  Includes index.
  1. Nursing schools—Faculty—Vocational guidance.
I. Title. [DNLM: 1. Education, Nursing. 2. Faculty,
Nursing. WY 19 Z28c]
RT90.Z36   1987   610.73′07′11   87-27099
ISBN 0-8385-1080-9

Designer: Steven M. Byrum
Production Editor: Charles F. Evans

PRINTED IN THE UNITED STATES OF AMERICA

Contributors

Gail C. Davis, Ed.D., R.N.
Associate Professor
College of Nursing
Texas Christian University
Fort Worth, Texas

Alice LeVeille Gaul, Ph.D., R.N.
Assistant Professor
College of Nursing
Texas Christian University
Fort Worth, Texas

Patricia D. Scearse, D.N.Sc., R.N.
Professor and Dean
College of Nursing
Texas Christian University
Fort Worth, Texas

Carol A. Stephenson, Ed.D., R.N.
Associate Professor
College of Nursing
Texas Christian University
Fort Worth, Texas

Margaret Denise Zanecchia, Ph.D., R.N.
Associate Professor
College of Nursing
Texas Christian University
Fort Worth, Texas

To my husband Joseph for his loving support: thank you.

            MDZ

Contents

Preface xi

Acknowledgments xiii

1 Interacting System Model 1
   Margaret Denise Zanecchia, Ph.D., R.N.

2 Roles and Responsibilities 15
   Margaret Denise Zanecchia, Ph.D., R.N.

3 Teaching and Service 39
   Alice LeVeille Gaul, Ph.D., R.N.

4 Practice, Education, and Research 57
   Gail C. Davis, Ed.D., R.N.

5 Productivity and Workloads 81
   Margaret Denise Zanecchia, Ph.D., R.N.

6 Career Entry 111
   Margaret Denise Zanecchia, Ph.D., R.N.

7 Rewards and Risks 133
   Patricia D. Scearse, D.N.Sc., R.N.

8 Career Management 149
   Margaret Denise Zanecchia, Ph.D., R.N. and Carol A. Stephenson, Ed.D., R.N.

9 Forecasting Future Careers 191
   Margaret Denise Zanecchia, Ph.D., R.N.

Index 213

Preface

The focus of *Career Guide for Nurse Educators* is the philosophical and pragmatic review of the issues relevant to the professional roles and responsibilities of the nurse educator in the college setting. The book is intended as a useful handbook for faculty, teachers, and potential teachers of nursing, and is designed as an easy reading guide to be used throughout each phase of the nurse educator's experience.

The goal of the text is to enable the nurse educator to: (1) select and enter the teaching community as a well-informed applicant–participant; (2) assume roles and responsibilities related both to the teaching position and to the teaching–learning environment; and (3) move toward self-actualization in a successful career in teaching.

Using a systems approach, the focus of this book is the nurse educator who enters the college system as a faculty member and who must make many decisions that affect the progress towards a successful career in teaching. Intersystem linkages among the educational system and the student, faculty, and curriculum subsystems are explained. The nurse educator faces these situations daily in academia.

Based on the open system concept, the Interacting System Model (ISM) for the nurse educator is presented. The ISM, representing open relationships between the educator and the learning environment, serves as the organizing framework for the book and is discussed in Chapter 1.

Chapter 2, Roles and Responsibilities, provides a compendium of information about the nature and scope of the multiple roles, relationships, and responsibilities of nurse educators in the college or university setting.

In Chapter 3, Teaching and Service, the classroom and clinical settings for teaching are described. Emphasis is on the teaching–learning process.

Practice, education, and research roles of the faculty are described in Chapter 4. Included are joint appointments, consultation, and faculty practice models.

Chapter 5 discusses productivity and workloads of nurse educators. The chapter includes faculty workload segments from a national survey by the author.

Career Entry, Chapter 6, deals with the position of the nurse educator from search through acceptance of the position.

In Chapter 7, the rewards and risks inherent in the role are analyzed including the basis of merit.

Chapter 8, Career Management, involves planning, development, and evaluation of the role as a nursing faculty. Reappointment, tenure, and promotion are reviewed.

The final chapter, Chapter 9, forecasts future careers in nursing education from the issues influencing the nurse educator's role in society. The chapter includes a survey, by the author, of nursing educators from member programs of the American Association of Colleges of Nursing who ranked the forces affecting nursing education.

From career selection and preparation through career changes, tenure, and retirement, the author examines the major phases in the role of the professional nurse educator. Characteristics of nurse educators, job descriptions, tasks, productivity, workloads, rewards, and occupational risks are the subjects featured.

There is a large body of literature concerning the preparation of teachers, but existing resources do not bring together the major functional components of the career of nurse educator in higher educational institutions. This book is intended to serve primarily as a resource and guide for beginning or seasoned teachers of nursing and for those nurses in a different functional role who are considering changing to a teaching career. Portions of the text are derived from experiences in clinical practice, teaching, and administration, and provide for delineation of present and future professional tasks of nurse educators.

The personal satisfactions to be derived from effective instruction, whatever the setting, be it classroom or clinical laboratory, are enhanced by an understanding of the impact of the teacher on the environment, and vice versa. There is a need for a balance between the faculty's preparation, expectations of the role, and the multiple tasks and responsibilities that are a part of the actual role of the nurse educator. This guide assists the nurse educator to assess individual career goals and predict potential issues of future concern to nursing education.

In addition, the text provides practical information for nurse educators who are changing career settings. Guidelines and suggestions for making these transitions give additional insights for understanding the socialization or resocialization process. Other professional educators may find the book to be a helpful tool when career change is indicated, but the guide will best serve the potential nurse faculty, the new faculty, and the experienced nursing faculty.

MDZ

Acknowledgments

I am very grateful to Dr. Janice E. Hayes, formerly Professor of Nursing at the University of Connecticut, for the confidence she had in me. Without her support, this project would never have been initiated.

My sincere thanks are extended to my senior editor, Charles Bollinger, for his encouragement in the earlier stages, and to Marion Kalstein-Welch, Executive Editor, during the later stages for her kindness and patience.

I also want to thank my dean, Dr. Patricia Scearse, for her chapter contribution, but more for the guidance necessary to make the completion of this book a reality.

I am especially indebted to my faculty colleagues, Dr. Gail Davis, Dr. Alice Gaul, and Dr. Carol Stephenson, who provided support for contributing chapters. Without them, the completion of this book would not have been possible.

My typist Peggy Sturgill deserves a special recognition and praise.

To each of you, my most sincere thanks.

MDZ

1

Interacting System Model

Margaret Denise Zanecchia, Ph.D., R.N.

In the past decades, the nursing profession has been faced with many tasks. Defining itself, asserting independence, and describing the levels of practice are a few of these tasks. Those involved in nursing education have been exploring appropriate educational preparation for students. Insufficient time has elapsed to build a research base to validate the problems that could possibly be contributing to the issues or to prescribe solutions. The changing health care system emerged with demands for professional nurses who were educated to meet the current and future needs (Grace, 1983).

The information age and the high-risk technological environment dictate the need for many nursing career patterns. For some, planning for a career that will span the nineties and serve the next century is critical. Economic restraints and supply–demand formulas affecting careers exist in the academic marketplace, the hospital, and the community. The availability of choices creates a situation of paramount importance for both the younger and older person beginning a career or considering a career change.

ACADEMIC PROFESSION

Nursing education is a growing academic profession. An *academic profession* is an occupational group of faculty dedicated to a specific discipline who exercise scholarly activities, the core of which is the advancement of knowledge. Nursing educators demonstrate a dyad in role: that of the professional nurse and the professional teacher.

Nursing faculty as autonomous professionals possess all the characteristics of a profession (Light, 1974, p. 11):

- Power to recruit and train new faculty members
- Power to judge who is qualified to have an academic appointment
- Responsibility to regulate the quality of the faculty's workload
- Ability to enjoy social prestige
- Responsibility to generate a body of knowledge

The college or university is generally accepted as the setting that best supports the education of a professional disciplinarian. In nursing, as in other scientific disciplines, the clinical learning laboratory enables nursing students to learn and practice. Innovative teaching strategies and newer classroom settings in the community are now in demand. The faculty develops a curriculum to teach the future students.

The nurse educator's role is a recurring series of activities; teaching is just one of them. To prepare nurse educators as clinical generalists and specialists who can teach additional clinical generalists and specialists to give highly technical care is a quest. Challenging students to think and to inquire and to conduct research is included in this role. The advancement of knowledge is the academic professional's ultimate concern (Dill, 1982).

MODELS

Models provide a way to look at something to make it more useful and easier to understand. A model is designed to explain an idea or to simplify a complex idea (Dickoff, James, & Weidenbach, 1968).

A *model* is a picture of selected parts. The parts are symbols of elements perceived to be the important phenomena involved (Stevens, 1979). The model reflects the relationships among the parts to explain the reason for the concept. Models based on theories serve as useful mechanisms for understanding and clarifying the more complicated situations.

Systems Model

In the past, *General Systems Theory* has been used to explain the many aspects of nursing and health care delivery. The basic systems model was defined by von Bertalanffy, and included structure, process, outcome, and a feedback loop. General Systems Theory was based on the science of wholeness or a set of components interacting with one another within boundaries. Systems involve both structure and process functions. The structure of a system was conceptualized by the arrangement of the system's parts, while the process was the dynamic change that occurred in the matter–energy characterizing the system (von Bertalanffy, 1968, p. 38).

In an open system, *input* is any measurable event or series of events outside the system, which enters and influences system output. *Output* expresses a product export, which can be detected and evaluated for reference. Reorganization and transformation of input within the system is known as *throughput* (Bertrand, 1972).

Nursing has used systems theory to effectively explain nursing theory, nursing process, and client care outcomes. The nursing process has also explored concepts to promote understanding about the phenomena within nursing.

A *system,* defined by Bevis (1978, p. 141), is the operational design of a process for achieving a specific purpose. In nursing education, the system's outputs are the outcomes of the learning. More specifically, the nurse educator (system input) interacts with the student or client to produce a form of outcome (the learning).

Interaction Model

In addition to the systems model, concepts of nursing, man, health, and environment have been viewed through models, which were behavioral, biological, developmental, eclectic, or interactional (Thibodeau, 1983, pp. 53–54). *Interaction* is seen by King (1971) as the interfacing of individuals in existential moments for some purpose or goal. *Transactions* are viewed as exchanges of energy and information among the persons involved in an interaction, which results in goal attainment. The interacting nursing model of King contains the elements of action, reaction, and transaction and uses the key terms of *personal system, interpersonal system,* and *social system.*

The total person was considered an open system in interaction with a total environment (Walker & Avant, 1983, p. 27). The nurse educator in every system is also affected by the total environment. Neuman (1980, pp. 119–125) conceptualized a health care systems model as a total-person approach to the client's problem. The nursing profession is a complete system with its own interrelating smaller systems, parts, and subparts. Nursing education and nursing practice would be examples of smaller whole systems, but within the larger system of nursing they are also subsystems.

Interacting System Model

The *Interacting System Model* (ISM) is a guide for the nurse educator in the college system. The conceptualization of the model derives from system theory and interactive theory. Structure, process, and outcome are the interactive phases of the ISM (Fig. 1–1).

The ISM provides an organizing framework for the nurse educator in the college system. The model depicts the organization of the college system as structure, process, and outcome components influenced by the environmental forces and modified through the feedback loop. The components of the college system are:

- Input (structure)
- Processes
- Output (outcomes)
- Environment (forces)
- Feedback

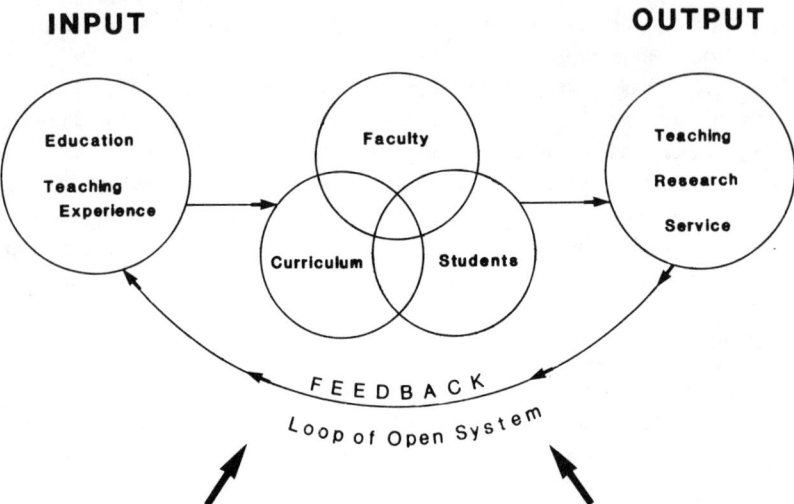

Figure 1-1. Interacting System Model. (*Courtesy of Margaret Denise Zanecchia, copyright 1987.*)

The career choice of an academic professional in nursing involves motivation, time, financial resources, and energy. The decision for a career as a nurse educator involves a dual commitment: to the profession of nursing and to the profession of teaching. A series of logical and planned steps is important and critical to the potential success of the individual nurse faculty member. The principal objective is a smooth transition into the pursuit of a career role as a faculty member. From the preparation for the role through the processes of the academic system, the potential nurse faculty system interacts in the college or university system.

INPUT STRUCTURE

The nurse educator enters the college system as a potential faculty member. The input or professional structure of the nurse educator is made up of educational degrees, certificates, and experience. The complete structure of the nurse educator is the total sum of the personal structure, including goals and ideals, with the professional structure.

Personal Structure
- Demographics
    Age
    Gender
    Economic status
    Ethnic background
- Health status
- Competencies

- Self-determination
- Motivation
- Personal characteristics
- Degree of self-satisfaction
- Goals
- Ideals

Professional Structure
- Degrees
- Experience

Nurse educators as input in the academic setting also may bring specialties and practitioner skills that will further extend their structure. A nurse faculty member may be prepared as a:

- Pediatric nurse practitioner
- Family nurse practitioner
- Geriatric nurse practitioner
- Psychiatric nurse clinician
- Adult nurse practitioner
- Nurse anesthetist
- Adolescent nurse clinician
- Nurse midwife

The current concept within the profession is the inclusion of specialty programs within a Master of Science in Nursing program, although this is not the case in all programs.

To be one who imparts knowledge is to seek and have knowledge. Nursing faculty continue to learn. Use of computer-assisted methodologies in teaching is a newer strategy. Computer literacy is implied with the future health care issues and cost containment. Nursing faculty are needed who can manage multiclient services throughout the community and model these skills for students.

The structure of the nurse educator, then, is that of an individual with a unique but complex personal and professional self. The elements of the structure have the potential to interact and influence the interaction of the faculty at any point upon entry into the system. The continuous interaction of the elements internal to the educator affects the entry processes and outcomes of the system (Cox, 1982, pp. 41–55). The nurse educator is depicted as formally entering the academic system when the pursuit of a faculty position results in a position.

PROCESS

The current model conceptualizes the college as the system. The individual is appointed to a faculty position in the system. From career entry through career goal achievements, the nurse educator interacts with the college system and multiple subsystems. Through the various processes, the nurse educator interacts with students, faculty, and the curriculum.

Once in the system and a part of the system's processes, the nurse educator interacts within three primary subsystems:

- Faculty subsystem
- Student subsystem
- Curriculum subsystem

Faculty Subsystem

The nurse educator in the college interacts in several subsystems, but for a faculty member, the faculty subsystem is primary. The faculty member in the faculty system is surrounded by the total college or university and the vast network of social systems of the outside community.

College and community social systems sometimes act as forces in the environment. Societal needs for production, reproduction, consumption, recreation, and education are met within the faculty subsystem, which is similar in function to the larger college and university systems.

The faculty subsystem is considered as both an independent and a dependent unit. It survives and maintains itself but cannot exist independently of the larger college system. Effective faculty–colleague–administrative interactions are necessary to maintain the faculty subsystem.

Input, process, output, and feedback first take place within the faculty subsystem. The faculty subsystem is supportive and has opportunity for reaction and interaction. It offers assisted actions on behalf of the faculty group. Meeting the faculty system's needs through a dynamic exchange is one of the interventions basic to the survival of the faculty system in many academic settings.

Each individual faculty member is a member of some type of faculty subsystem constellation, small or large, simple or complex. Although nursing faculty exist for the purpose of teaching students, at the same time they are concerned about their own functions and environment.

Faculty and faculty subsystems interact with the forces of the environment. These interactions have significant influence on the goals, objectives, and mission of the academic system. The promotion of student learning can be diminished or magnified by a dysfunctional faculty, or an environment not conducive to learning, or both.

Because the faculty subsystem is a unit, it also is a system. Smaller interdependent units of the faculty are composed of groups of faculty members. These configurations of units interact within the total faculty group, i.e., professional colleague groups and the personal social group. In these smaller groups, faculty go about the tasks necessary for the faculty subsystem to maintain itself and function. The committee is one example of a professional group interacting purposefully. The interacting framework of the social group is another example of these smaller faculty units. Personal and interpersonal relationships among faculty affect the goals of the faculty group.

Frequently, the neophyte nurse educator receives much less direct supervision than the new nurse in the clinical setting. The admission into an ongoing, organized subsystem, i.e., the faculty subsystem, and acceptance as a colleague requires much of the readjustment experienced as a new nurse in a practice setting (Jacox, 1982). The orientation at admission and adjustment by the new nurse educator can influence the prediction of success.

The university or college as a system has been well addressed in educational literature. However, the nature and effect of the complex interactions of the systems and subsystems within higher education have received little attention (Cohen & March, 1974; Baldridge, Curtis, Ecker, & Riley, 1978, p. 47). American higher education as a system describes the role of faculty in three major functions: teaching, research, and service. All of these functions or subsystems are no different for nursing than in other disciplines. The teaching–learning process and exchange of knowledge within the academic setting is usually considered the most important function. Practice in nursing may also be interpreted as a function, but means maintaining professional expertise.

Student Subsystem

The second primary subsystem in which the nurse educator interacts is the student subsystem. The student subsystem involves many complex internal subsystems. The smaller supporting systems or units of the student subsystem are necessary to assist students to maintain themselves in the learning environment.

The "college" experience includes learning beyond the traditional curriculum objectives into the development of a societal member, a citizen. Educational needs of students can be and are met informally through a variety of additional support systems such as extracurricular and social activities:

- Student recruiting
- Student big brothers–big sisters buddy system
- Registrar
- Student advisement
- Student work-study
- Student aid
- Data processing and computer center
- Food services
- Student health services
- Bookstore, materials, supplies
- Library services
- Recreation and sports
- Student counseling and tutoring
- Placement office
- Student newspaper, student radio and television station, communication system
- Security, protection, campus police
- Grievance and governance

All of the services required by the student subsystem must be coordinated with the curriculum and faculty subsystem. It is the function of college administration to monitor the interactive processes of all these smaller but vital systems dedicated to assisting the student in some way toward graduation.

The nurse educator interacts and interfaces with all of these support systems. Many of these activities use faculty supervision, which is necessary to assist the student to exit through the college system. Faculty may serve on committees to facilitate each of these activities.

Curriculum Subsystem

Of the three subsystems for the nurse faculty, the largest and most complex in which the nursing faculty interacts is the curriculum subsystem. As in the faculty and student subsystems, the curriculum subsystem has many smaller units supporting the larger system.

The unique units of the curriculum subsystem include:

- Course offerings
- Course crediting allowance
- Grading system
- Schedule of courses
- Class ranking
- Level of course
- Graduation requirements
- Degree plan
- Awards and honors

The curriculum is usually composed of courses of study. The curriculum has a core of general education courses. The courses in nursing or the specialization make up the major.

The general education curriculum has been regarded as a base or a foundation on which is built the student's content focus, nursing. The curriculum subsystem is a plan, which provides sets of learning opportunities for students so they may achieve educational goals related to specific learning objectives. The subsystem of the curriculum provides the foundational process of the teaching–learning process in a particular institution.

The nurse educator guides students through the total curriculum in order to assist them in the achievement of successful outcomes. This assistance is known as the *advisement process*. The nurse educator's role is to advise the student on the general and specialized components of the curriculum and to facilitate the selection and succession of courses.

OUTCOMES AND OUTPUTS

For a student, the major outcomes of learning include graduation, college degrees, career preparation, self-satisfaction, and future employment (Astin, 1977, p. 7).

Examples of student nurse outputs include: degrees, licensure as a professional nurse, more knowledge, potential employment, self-fulfillment, and social change. The output increases with larger numbers of students who graduate or are granted college degrees. Other student outputs are higher than average grade point at graduation, higher class rank, awards and honors.

Faculty Outputs

The output of the college system is both student-related and faculty-related. As the faculty performs its roles, i.e., teaching, research, and service, the objectives of the system are met and goals achieved.

Outcomes of the faculty are primarily the learning of the students, but faculty output also includes increased knowledge about nursing, publications, research, practice, service, and grants. Outcomes for nursing faculty are creative instructional materials, the products of research, and service. Outcomes for faculty also include: increased teaching skills, an increased knowledge about nursing, social change, increased practice capabilities, more research conducted, higher publication rate, more funded grants, accredited programs, and awards.

The measures of output from the nurse educator in the practice role are more difficult to assess, but improved health states for students or clients could be demonstrated through the evaluation of selected statistics collected on the population. For example, the client group may have a:

- Decrease in number of motor vehicle accidents
- Decreased morbidity
- Lowered infant mortality rates
- Increased passing scores on client health knowledge quizzes
- Changes in eating behaviors toward a balanced diet intake
- Weight loss of obese clients
- Decreased numbers in recalcitrant clinic visits
- More early cancer diagnoses
- Increased number of immunizations
- Decreased absenteeism in schools

The measures of nurse educator output for the faculty group may also include the above as well as more informed faculty peers of the faculty subsystem.

Feedback

Whatever does happen in the system and during the interactive process between the faculty, the students, and the curriculum, the interaction will always have substantial impact on the outcome. Feedback is essential.

The economic demands, which have been placed on the educational system, require demonstrations of productivity. Modification is necessary, and substantial changes in any or all of the subsystems may be required. Through the feedback loop, the input (structure) processes and output (outcomes) are modified to better achieve the system's goals.

The evaluation process is the mechanism for assessing outcomes. The usual method by which the nurse educator in any system can determine how or if a change in the system output should take place is by assessing whether the system's objectives are being met. Evaluation should be objective, well documented, measurable, systematized, and based on standards and criteria.

A major problem in health care settings, according to Mauksch and Miller (1981), is the discontinuation of change based on emotional rather than objective data. The feedback mechanisms of open college systems provide the means to improve the processes that may need changing to better accomplish the goals of the system. Feedback can also lead to evaluative changes and reorganization of the system itself.

Environmental Forces

Interlinking and interrelating forces affect the function of the total system. External environment subsystem forces control the processes of the system. Networking, mentoring, and research can be utilized for the purpose of feedback and as recognition of and sensitivity to newer external subsystems. Nursing faculty and education monitor the effect of these moral, social, political, or economic forces on the total system.

The most important of the external forces acting on the system are human and economic resources. Human resources consist of personnel (administrative, peers, and subordinates). Persons at all levels interact with the nurse educator and may serve as weak or strong, positive or negative stressors. Professional personnel and clients are two of the largest groups of resources within the nursing education system. Within the environment external to the total system, other groups of persons (i.e., unions, professional organizations, accreditation bodies, and society's consumers) act as forces impacting on the nursing education system.

The mission, goals, and financial management of the individual college, hospital, or community agency educator are to be considered as external forces by the nurse educator. Within the organization are inherent program costs and economics relevant to the control of budget, materials, facilities, resources, and the quota of nursing educators. The forces of several subsystems, internal and external, also affect the number of nursing educational systems and budget spending. Internal subsystems include the number of student clients, curriculum programs, and administrative expectations for the faculty.

Subsystem interactions potentiate actions while generating reactions and integration concurrently within the individual nurse educator. The processes of these subsystems affect the individual nurse educator's intrapersonal, interpersonal, and extrapersonal systems. Effects of these forces also have potential to change the outcomes of the very system or the subsystems on which they act. While the forces may bring about positive or negative output from the system, a strong desire to control the forces exists within and outside the nursing profession. Feedback mechanisms are necessary to bring the forces within a controllable range so the system may profit without danger of interruption or an untoward total system change.

Society's need for nurses and nurse educators is a constant force dictating the demand for type and numbers of nurses. The nursing profession itself is a strong external system that affects the nursing education system and the total educational system. Nursing and nursing education exert control on the structure, process, and outcome and on the goals and objectives of the nursing educational system.

The college is viewed as an open dynamic system according to Richman and Farmer (1974). The college interacts with multiple internal and external subsystems beyond those of the faculty, students, and curriculum. Regardless of the mission, goals, or objectives of the college system, the college also interacts within an environment and a vast number of external forces. These forces are important sources of power, which influence the college educational system. How the college changes input into output is influenced by forces and sources of power. Outcome prediction and testing of outcome theory will involve the research efforts of nurses in higher education in future years.

SUMMARY

Whatever the institutional climates and forces, the morale of the college system and the faculty are affected. The nurse educator should become aware of the institutional characteristics so that a match between personal goals and institutional mission can be found. Studies of perceived and preferred goals in educational institutions have identified academic freedom, an inquiry approach, research, academic development, and an intellectual environment as being among those qualities of an institution that faculty consider of major importance in consideration of academic employment (Peterson & Uhl, 1977, pp. 63–67).

According to Pace (1979, p. 163), the direction for the future will be to find the commonalities involved in educational institutions between outcomes and goals of the faculty and the student outcomes and achievement.

Systems theory and interacting theory have been successfully utilized in the past to explicate the art and science of nursing. Systems theory when applied to the college provides an operative method through which nursing practice is measured. Several nursing models have been designed and implemented. Models strengthen nursing practice and serve the professional nursing system through confirmation of scientific principles, concepts, processes, and rationale.

In an application of systems theory, health organizations have been described by Georgopolous (1966, p. 12) as complex, sociotechnical systems with inputs of raw materials, supplies, personnel, skills, and attitudes and a primary output of quality of care. He believed that there were critical processes of resource allocation, control, coordination of effort, social and psychological integration, organizational strain, and management between the inputs and the outputs. All of these forces have the potential to interact and to modify the relationships of the nurse educators with the variables and outcomes of the system.

Though nursing is an independent and interdependent profession, various collaborative relationships exist and affect the output. In every system and subsystem of the college, nurse educators function with both health- and nonhealth-related professional personnel. While a nurse's primary goals include assisting clients to attain or maintain optimum wellness, the nurse educator's goals are to teach students to deliver knowledgeable quality care to clients. A healthier community-at-large and a more informed consumer client are among the desired professional outcomes of the college system.

Society as a whole gains from the production of learning and the possibility for the development of the full potentiality of human beings. When the teacher has imparted knowledge to the formative student mind, great personal satisfaction is experienced. The nurse educator who has met these challenges will find congruent records and career satisfaction in the college setting.

Quality of the educational product is reflected in the outcomes of the system, which provided it. The Interacting System Model (ISM) for the nurse educator in the college system purports to measure outcomes of the student subsystem (i.e., graduation, degrees, professional licensure), and the faculty subsystem (i.e., quality teaching, research, publications, and service). Outcomes achieved through the systems' processes are evaluated and modified (feedback) for change and improvement to better meet the needs of society's consumers of nursing.

As nursing faculty (structure or input) characteristics such as educational background and professional experience change, the processes of the college system and subsystems may change. The outputs (products) of individual faculty and faculty as a group are influenced by the functions of the interactive system. Many dynamic environmental forces (society, politics, economics, supply and demand) regulate the system.

In the ISM, college outcomes affect mainly two groups: students and faculty. Outcomes or output in systems terms reflect what is produced following the interacting processes of the system, subsystems, and internal forces. Output from any system is formally or informally evaluated through feedback and may be modified. External forces in the environment act to change and influence the system.

The major types of output that can be produced through the interacting of the three subsystems are student centered and faculty centered. The nurse educator in the college system has a greater or lesser role in the productivity of the outputs depending on the system, subsystems, complexity of smaller units, openness, environmental forces or restraints, and feedback.

Nursing educators must assume accountability for providing students not only with a quality education, but with the kind of education that challenges them to generate theory as a basis for the domain of nursing practice. When the commitment for quality assurance in nursing education is a part of the inherited endowment, desired outcomes for professional nursing can be achieved (Moore, Damewood, & Jewell, 1984).

The health care model of the future will be comprehensive, preventative, collaborative, and community-based, and it should be designed for clients of all ages, developmental stages, races, socioeconomic levels, and health states. The care of clients in the future will be affected by the students of today, who will be their professional caregivers.

REFERENCES

Astin, A. (1977). *Four critical years* (pp. ix, 7). San Francisco: Jossey-Bass Publishers.
Baldridge, J. V., Curtis, D. V., Ecker, G., & Riley, G. L. (1978). *Policy making and effective leadership* (p. 47). San Francisco: Jossey-Bass Publishers.
Bertrand, A. (1972). *Social organization: A general system and role theory perspective* (pp. 91–105). Philadelphia: F. A. Davis.
Bevis, E. (1978). *Curriculum building in nursing* (p. 141). St. Louis: C. V. Mosby.
Cohen, M., & March, J. (1974). *Leadership and ambiguity: The American college president.* New York: McGraw-Hill.
Cox, C. (1982). An interaction model of client health behavior: Theoretical prescription for nursing. *Advances in Nursing Science, 1*(5), 41–55.
Dickoff, J., James, P., & Weidenbach, E. (1968). Theory in a practice discipline. *Nursing Research, 17,* 415–435.
Dill, D. D. (1982). The structure of the academic profession. *Journal of Higher Education, 53*(3), 255–267.
Georgopolous, B. (1966). The hospital system and nursing: Some basic problems and issues. *Nursing Forum, 5*(3), 8–35.
Grace, H. (1983). In C. McGuire, R. Foley, A. Gore, & R. Richards (Eds.), *Handbook of health professions education* (pp. 92–110). San Francisco: Jossey-Bass Publishers.
Jacox, A. (1982). Prerequisites for the exercise of professionalism. *Briefly Noted: Literary Soaps for Deans, 2*(2), Viewpoints #8.
King, I. (1971). *Toward a theory of nursing.* New York: John Wiley & Sons.
Light, D. (1974). Introduction: The structure of the academic profession. *Sociology of Education, 47,* 2–28.
Mauksch, I., & Miller, M. (1981). *Implementing change in nursing* (pp. 148–149). St. Louis: C. V. Mosby Co.
Moore, L., Damewood, C. F., & Jewell, K. (1984). A method for achieving quality assurance in nursing education. *Nursing & Health Care, 5*(5), 269–274.
Neuman, B. (1980). The Betty Neuman health-care systems model: A total person approach to patient problems. In J. Riehl & C. Roy (Eds.), *Conceptual models for nursing practice* (2nd ed.) (pp. 119–125). New York: Appleton-Century-Crofts.
Pace, C. (1979). *Measuring outcomes of college* (p. 163). San Francisco: Jossey-Bass Publishers.
Peterson, R., & Uhl, N. (1977). *Formulating college and university goals: A guide for using the institutional goals inventory* (pp. 63–67). Princeton, New Jersey: Educational Testing Service.
Richman, B., & Farmer, R. (1974). *Leadership, goals and power in higher education.* San Francisco: Jossey-Bass Publishers.
Stevens, B. J. (1979). *Nursing theory: Analysis application evaluation.* Boston: Little, Brown.
Thibodeau, J. (1983). *Nursing models: Analysis and evaluation* (pp. 53–54). Monterey, Calif.: Wadsworth Health Science Division.
von Bertalanffy, L. (1968). *General systems theory* (p. 38). New York: George Braziller, Inc.
Walker, L., & Avant, K. (1983). *Strategies for theory construction in nursing* (p. 27). E. Norwalk, Conn.: Appleton-Century-Crofts.

2

Roles and Responsibilities

Margaret Denise Zanecchia, Ph.D., R.N.

The emphasis of professional nursing has changed from direct caregiving to clients more towards the facilitating of a care and self-care model. The role of nursing education is also changing. While consumerism exists in the academic marketplace, the emphasis in nursing education has shifted from the teacher and the teaching process to the learner and the learning process.

The Interacting System Model (ISM) provides a flexible open framework through which learning may be viewed as the outcome of the college or university system. Teaching and student learning are the primary objectives for the nurse educator. The objectives are measurable and derive from the stated mission and philosophy of the institution.

Traditionally, the institution of higher learning has a threefold mission: the acquisition of knowledge, or research; the transmission of knowledge, or teaching; and the application of knowledge, which is community service (Rustia, 1983a, pp. 66–71). Nurse educators may prefer one of the role activities—teaching, research, or service—more than another. If so, an attempt to find the best setting and role is suggested. Then faculty members may have some assurance that teaching, research, or service activities prevail.

The philosophy, objectives, kinds of students, and conditions of employment also may vary in different kinds of nursing education programs. Nurse educators seeking employment may make a preliminary assessment of an educational program and setting. It is important to identify the philosophy of the institution and the program as being congruent with the philosophy of the nurse educator (Kelly, 1981a, p. 298). One can function more effectively when setting, activities, and personal philosophy are compatible.

The nurse educator simultaneously performs as a professional nurse and as a teacher. As an educator, the nurse brings a unique personal philosophy to the role. The philosophical basis of the professional nurse educator's role encompasses a joint philosophy of nursing and education. The successful teacher believes the student will and can learn. Many theories of education exist and are utilized in nursing education. Whatever the theories of teaching–learning, the nurse educator's philosophy of education greatly affects the teaching role and, consequently, the student's learning.

The nurse educator's philosophy of nursing also affects the teaching role. Throughout the years, the emphasis on well-informed consumers through client health teaching expands the teaching role of the nurse. Because the nursing faculty member is first of all a nurse, the unique belief about nursing as an art and a science affects the teaching. The nurse educator practices and teaches within the dimensions of a personal philosophy of nursing. The early socialization of the professional nurse affects the integration of the roles of the dyad as professional nurse and educator (Fagin & McGivern, 1983, p. 212).

The roles, relationships, and responsibilities of the nurse educator are multiple, complex, and incorporate a multitude of tasks. The nurse educator functions in various roles within the many systems and subsystems of all college systems and subsystems and in various settings: classroom, college laboratory, clinical laboratory, and the community at large. Some roles are common to certain settings, but the primary roles of teaching, research, and service exist in the college setting.

Unlimited types and numbers of relationships are apparent in all teaching settings between students, nurse educators, administrators, peers, and the clients of students. A variety of teaching styles, personalities, and presentations of instruction are found within all settings (Eble, 1973, p. 170). A great potential for dynamic relationships with many groups is challenging for educators in the college-setting role.

Academic roles are becoming more diffuse and more difficult to identify. Multiple requirements beyond the demands of traditional teaching, research, and service have evolved. In classroom and laboratory settings, the roles of the nursing faculty involve multiple tasks, responsibilities, and expectations. As in any profession, a need for planning and scheduling necessary activities is required to accomplish the tasks. When realistic goals and identified priorities are set, the effectiveness of the tasks performed can be evaluated (Charron, 1985, pp. 77–79).

The typical responsibilities of the position of nurse educator are those required to accomplish the objectives of measurable student learning and published discoveries of knowledge. While teaching is the primary role of the nurse educators in the college system, research and service further expand the role. But regardless of the setting, all of the activities included in the role of the nurse educator are potentially dynamic, potentially innovative, and challenging.

Similar to higher education, the three standard role activities of the nursing faculty are historically teaching, research, and service. In the past, the time and effort spent on these tasks was given priority, although teaching claimed more of the faculty's time and energy than the other two. If all the tasks were effectively accomplished, the nurse educator met the requirements of the position, fulfilled the role, and earned the rewards.

According to Dressel and Mayhew (1974, p. 332), most faculty engage in certain common activities. Among the activities are instruction, preparation of curriculum, advising, research and scholarly activity, professional service, and participation in governance at the departmental, college, and university level. Faculty with different levels of expertise, interest, and motivation may perform selected activities. The choice of these activities affects the faculty role. Often faculty constitute a role according to individual expertise. Some perform the roles that are more comfortable. The nurse educator, as a faculty member, has functioned in the role of an academic professional through a recurring series of activities (Dill, 1982, p. 260).

The activities of the nursing role can be grouped into two types of task groups: the major role tasks and the related role tasks.

ROLES OF THE NURSING FACULTY

Major Roles
- Teaching
- Research
- Service
- Advising
- Curriculum development
- Clinical practice

Student-related Roles
- Recruiter
- Advocate
- Preceptor
- Tutor

Faculty-related Roles
- Administrative governance
- Professional organization member
- Education provider-consumer
- Political leader
- Mentor

As previously stated, the major role tasks consume most of the nurse educator's time and effort. An outstanding performance on these tasks gains the highest rewards of the academic system.

The related role tasks include a variety of less important but necessary activities, which are required for the operation of the college system as an institution of higher learning. These activities are categorized according to the group in which the faculty is more involved.

MAJOR ROLES

Teaching

Teaching is the main responsibility of the nurse educator. Teaching is described as the greatest of all tasks (Schweer, 1968, p. 39). Good teaching is the expectation of any institution of higher learning, whether it occurs in the classroom or the laboratory. The reputation of being an excellent teacher is one of the coveted rewards to be earned by any faculty, including the nursing faculty. Once earned, it is re-earned through a continuing series of activities.

Teaching includes the instruction of undergraduate, graduate, and doctoral students. Instruction includes preparation of the instructional materials and the evaluation and grading of the students' progress. The challenge of teaching is to motivate the student to learn and to facilitate the learning.

The student's learning should be organized, sequenced, and supervised by the instructor so that new knowledge and skills are consistently gained. As part of the role, the nurse educator provides both meaningful materials and clinical experiences for students. The teaching of students includes a comprehensive evaluation of performance on which students are informed.

The teaching–instructing role is divided between two settings, the classroom and the clinical area. Both settings have characteristics that influence the teaching role: organizational elements, physical facilities, time of day, day of the week, number of students, and content (Dixon, 1977, p. 59). The nurse educator remains flexible and adapts the teaching to a number of characteristics.

Heidgerken (1965, p. 33) states that the functions of the role of teaching are constantly changing because the foundations of knowledge keep growing and the demands (i.e., new technology and increased responsibilities) are continually being added to the knowledge base. This is even more true today as technology expands at a quickening pace. Because nursing is an academic discipline and a professional practice discipline, the scientific discoveries must be taught within the art of nursing and integrated into the total curriculum. Teaching students about the health care of clients must be a continuous process.

The nurse educator's role as a teacher can potentially influence the total nursing profession towards a more autonomous and actualized state (Weiss, 1984). Nursing deans are needed whose leadership can inspire nurse educators. Creative designs and implementation of quality nursing programs will assist students in becoming autonomous professionals (Van Ort, 1985, p. 236). Nurse educators comprise the group that influences the future nursing profession.

Research

University teaching and research complement each other. Through teaching, educators reveal unsolved problems yet to be studied. Research or the discoveries of knowledge is shared by educators with their students (Vemulapalli, 1984).

The meaning of the research role is broad and encompasses the pursuit of knowledge through scholarly activities. Scholarly pursuits resulting in publications are the strongest evidence to evaluate the research skill of the faculty. The expectation of continued research publication in refereed journals in one's area of specialization is a criterion documenting continued competence (Schurr, 1982, p. 330).

The purposes of research in the college setting are (1) to improve teaching and the curriculum, and (2) to produce knowledge and problem solving (Dressel, 1978, pp. 360–361). Faculty at all levels engage in some research to be considered productive in the role of an educator. Research is a newer expectation for the nurse educator in the college system.

In fact, the nurse educator's role in the college demands research. As researchers, nurses need to explain, predict, and control phenomena, which are within the scope of nursing (Hollshwandnen, Kinney & Paradowski, 1984, p. 144). The research task includes design of research studies, creating grants, scholarly activities, publication of the findings of scientific study, and invited presentations at national and international conferences.

The definition of scholarly activity in nursing was the subject of a national survey in 1985 (Baird et al., 1985, p. 146). "Scholarly activity" was used synonymously with "research." Doctoral study, being a primary author of a book, writing a grant that is fundable, being a speaker at a national conference, and receiving a national professional award were used more often to identify scholarly activity. In addition to these, other important tasks, which defined scholarly activity, included: publishing research in a refereed journal, speaking to a regional or local group, presenting continuing education, writing a grant proposal, which was not funded, and publishing a theoretical article.

While scholarship is learning or knowledge acquired by study, Diers (1983, p. 3) found thinking to be a tool of clinical scholarship. Thinking, it was believed, could raise the conclusions from research to the level of implications, interpretation, concept, or theory.

The central concepts and themes of nursing are described as a metaparadigm of nursing. One of the goals for nurse researchers is the generation and testing of nursing theories (Fawcett, 1984, p. 87). Research activities can result in the production of new knowledge and in the development of theory. The post-1950 period has been a time of increased research productivity for nurse educators, but future research activities need to be directed toward building a science for nursing practice (Brown, Tanner, & Padrick, 1984, p. 31).

While theory development is another element of the research role of the nurse educator, inquiry into the phenomenon of nursing has generated some answers to practice questions. Practice-based research had provided a strong foundation for decisions that improve health care (Lancaster, 1984, p. 379). The nurse educator who is involved in clinical research has the potential to bridge the gap between education and service through collaborative models. Both a university- and an agency-based model have been successfully utilized for collaborative research (Loomis & Krone, 1980, pp. 32–35).

An important advantage of faculty research has been the stimulation of student learning through the faculty's enthusiasm for research. Students can learn by participating in research. Faculty members have stimulated one another to join in the creation of further research. Scholarly activity is an important criteria for evaluating the performance of the nurse educator.

Service

Service to the college has been described as all of the activities directed toward improving the operation of the college system. The service role for nursing faculty exists in the college setting and, historically, it has been one of the three major role tasks. The service role in the college, internal and external public service, is less well defined, but it involves interdepartmental, intradepartmental, and interagency services provided by the nurse educator.

Academic services are provided for the faculty of the college. Internal or on-campus service programs support the achievement of the basic purposes of instruction, research, and external service. Some examples of internal service are library, media support, computer services, and student development services.

In a macroperspective view, administration, financial affairs, development, operations, and the maintenance of the physical plant are internal services for the faculty (Dressel, 1978, pp. 365–366). Internal services activities include faculty members advising to other departments in the areas of their specializations (i.e., computer, research design, or test construction). Service roles provided by faculty include vocational and academic counseling and administrative committee work.

External services offered by faculty involve off-campus activities, i.e., cooperative extensions, continuing education, and consultative services for individuals and community groups. Assistance with research on community-based problems is considered an external service of the faculty. Other external services include roles such as editor, paper or proposal referee, paid consultant, voluntary consultant, institutional accreditation committee member, guest lecturer, convention attendee, expert witness, inventor, and part-time administrator (Scriven, 1982, p. 311).

Public service involves the nurse educator with social, business, governmental, and industrial groups of all types and at all levels. For example, some service contacts can generate sources for future clinical laboratory sites. Visibility may be attained with organizational representatives who may be responsible for financial support from benefactors. Increasing endowments, gifts, and scholarships for the nursing department or other departments in the institution can be a result of positive service exchanges between the college and the community.

The professional service activity has involved the nurse educator as a professional nurse in a direct nursing role. Usually, the nurse educator has performed some type of nursing activity as a compensated employee, but the activity could be performed in a voluntary capacity. The focus of the service to the profession is dedicated to the discipline of nursing as an organized group.

Local and regional contacts made through service and the accompanying travel can build a broader cadre of service relationships. As the exchanges increase between faculty and those served, productive national and international relationships can result.

Nursing faculties have made major contributions to the university's mission of service. The more typical services range from various screening clinics to needs surveys of elderly clients. Nursing clinics are established at schools of nursing. These clinics support student learning experiences and faculty practice endeavors. Other examples of community service have included parenting and childbirth classes (Andruskiw, 1983, pp. 15–16).

Joint community services successfully demonstrate collaboration between faculty from nursing schools and from schools of education and sociology (i.e., preschool programs). These combined efforts encourage and strengthen interdisciplinary relationships and support for nursing.

The service activities of the nurse educator in the college setting are coordinated within the mission of the institution. In addition to the teaching and the research roles, the service role is a measured outcome of the system. The service activities of the nurse educator are evaluated with the other role tasks.

Advising

Academic advising is providing educationally related information and guidance to students confronted with choices and alternative paths in the curriculum (Trombley & Holmes, 1980, p. 20). Some consider advising as a part of the curriculum development role, but most have agreed it is a separate part of the academic process.

Many other ancillary roles have been identified, and some have become a part of the role of advisor. According to Mayhew (1970), undergraduate students have needed some consistent personal contact with a professional adult who can serve as an advisor, confidant, and parent surrogate. Over the years both positive and negative opinions have existed regarding the acceptance of these ancillary advisor roles.

The three types of academic advising that involve nursing faculty are general advising, resource advising, and advising in the nursing major. A good advising system requires coordination between the faculty in the nursing department in addition to faculty and staff in all the other departments of the institution. Consistent and long-term efforts are necessary for a successful advising system.

The advising workload is shared with all faculty and in some programs with administration. The dean advises a small group in addition to those seen for special problems. The number of advisees fluctuates, but the average load ranges between 13 to 17 students per faculty member. Some institutions adjust the teaching assignment to support the advisement workload. Reduced teaching load and specific preparation for the advising role are suggested.

The advisor appointed for each nursing student is usually a nurse educator. The advisor is assigned to the student preferably very early in the program. Students remain within the same individual faculty for advisement until the student has graduated. However, because of faculty turnover, students may have a new advisor every year.

The requirements for a good advisor include a broad range of skills and knowledge, strong motivation and, in addition, large amounts of prescheduled and unscheduled or "open-door" time. Excellent communication skills and, more recently, computer skills are an asset. The most important characteristic is the ability of the faculty to understand students. Understanding the perceptions of students gives advisors the necessary insights into students' interactions. The quality of the advisor–advisee relationship has great influence on the student's continued and successful progress.

The faculty member who is a good advisor is a master of listening skills, in addition to all aspects of the curriculum: admission, registration, retention, and graduation requirements. This faculty advisor truly assists the student through the college system. Students ponder alternative methods to earn credit: work-study, challenging exams for credit, contracts, independent study, transfer courses, second degrees, minors, honors, and maybe more. The advantages and disadvantages of various paths through the curriculum and the course-by-course options are in the purview of the good nursing advisor.

Tailoring the available options for courses and the sequencing of courses to the individual students' needs and interests is the goal, according to Dressel (1978, p. 359). When a student advisement system was evaluated, a student wrote, "Please be helpful and encouraging when a student attempts to individualize her education." Another student cautioned, "Please be sure your information is correct" (Bossenmaier, 1979, pp. 787–791). The faculty person who has not learned the intricacies of the curriculum should seek the advice from those faculty members who are more experienced. With the high cost of education, students should not have to tolerate the results of inadequate or erroneous advisement. Academic advice when articulated by the faculty can have a binding effect upon the institution (Jones, 1983, p. 84).

Students have requested and needed assistance and guidance from faculty during hours when students are available. These periods may occur during lunchtime or at other times that are not as convenient for faculty. Students want the opportunity for informal contact and discussion of problems, courses, and career. It is not always feasible for students to make a formal appointment for advisement.

Outside of the actual class contact, faculty have less opportunity to interact with students. Through the advisement program, interest may be conveyed and an enthusiastic message of encouragement for the student's progress may be demonstrated. Sometimes students have also hoped to have a chance to talk about nursing with the faculty while not in a formal learning situation.

On the other side, nurse educators can learn to advise. Hopefully, the well-advised, satisfied students complete programs. Positive advising and high retention rates have been correlated with institutional goals and outcomes (Trombley & Holmes, 1980, pp. 20–24).

Occasionally, advising overlaps with counseling. Counseling becomes necessary for students who experience more serious problems. Personal problems that are causing stress for the student need attention. The inability to continue learning for any reason demands the assistance of a counselor. The role of the nurse educator is to refer the student to the college counseling center. Although many faculty assume the counseling role, it is better to refer the student for professional assistance.

Since the advising activity in the role of the nurse educator is difficult to define, it is also a problem to evaluate. As with teaching, advising does not offer the same type of rewards to faculty as the other major role tasks. However, advising is becoming more important for the nurse educator because of student consumerism. Declining enrollments mean fewer students and more need to give better advice. Because of this gain in importance in the college system, the nurse educator's role in advising is one of the major role tasks. Evaluation mechanisms for advisement productivity exist in some institutions.

Curriculum Development

In the Interacting System Model, the curriculum is a subsystem of the larger college system. The curriculum is affected by forces in the environment, society, the institution characteristics, the student group, and the design of the curriculum itself (Conrad & Pratt, 1983, pp. 23–24). In addition, all of the interrelationships among these forces and groups influence the development of curriculum through change in structure, process, outcome, or feedback of the system.

Generally, the content of the nursing curriculum is developed on the basis of the needs for practice and those of society's clients and employers (Reed, 1983, p. 157–165). The ISM depicts the social needs as forces in the environment, which also affect the nurse in the college classroom or clinical laboratory setting. Curriculum development in any setting, formal or informal, i.e., continuing education, follows the same process. When followed, a systematic process provides direction for further development, implementation, and evaluation (Wise, 1980, p. 318). Mechanisms for continuing modifications and updating of curricula are necessary.

Curricula are developed and described in a variety of ways: integrated, modularized, competency-based, research-based, articulated, holistic, technological, and humanistic. Elements of curricula are: philosophy, purpose, goals, conceptual framework, and multiple levels of measurable objectives. The curriculum for nursing programs usually is divided into lecture hours and clinical hours. Clinical agencies support the student laboratory experiences through the assignment of patient care (Lawrence & Lawrence, 1983, p. 163).

All curricula are evaluated by nursing faculty. The abilities of graduates demonstrate the educational outcomes of the curriculum. A demand for measurable results is a part of the mission and accountability of the college system. The role of the nurse educator is the development and implementation of a curriculum, which assists students in achieving outcomes.

Through the years, curricula in nursing programs have followed the medical model or one of the nursing models. The nurse educator's role in curriculum development, unlike the other major role tasks, is never completed. Due to the proliferation of knowledge, the universal access to information is more through computerization. The constantly changing technological environment requires curricula that need to be constantly re-examined (Sullivan & Brye, 1983, p. 187).

Nursing practice has demanded that nursing education be current to prepare students for the health care needs of the future client. Curriculum development should be ongoing, systematic, and based on the needs analysis. Curricula oriented toward the prevention of health problems and the maintenance of a healthy state in the community are more appropriate now (Sullivan & Brye, 1983, p. 187).

Curriculum development is affected by evaluation and is changed to meet consumer needs. The learning needs of students include intellectual, interpersonal, and technical skills. Core content for practice is necessary in acute and nonacute settings. Also, curriculum integrates the application of principles, concepts, and the nursing process (Schroeder, 1981, pp. 10–17). The role of the nurse educator includes research on curriculum. Changes can be based on facts.

Curriculum is developed to provide more opportunities for students to learn writing skills, critical thinking, clinical judgment, and decision making under faculty supervision (Pinkava & Haviland, 1984, pp. 270–272; Heckenberger, 1983, p. 181). One of the weaknesses identified in the nursing curriculum is the mechanism for the development of cognitive processes. Students who systematically organize and process task-related information are more able to integrate technical skills into patient care (Bolton, 1984, p. 385). The process-oriented curriculum is one possibility.

Many concerns have been expressed relative to the economic impact on health care of the baccalaureate nursing curriculum. However more costly, the nurse with a baccalaureate degree is needed to meet the new demand for professional health care. Cost–benefit studies that demonstrate improved delivery of nursing care could influence curriculum change (Stevens, 1985, p. 125). The challenge for the contemporary nurse educator is curriculum development for a program that produces a professional generalist who is more effective in delivering quality and quantity of care than others who cannot. The approach to care is different for the baccalaureate nurse.

Clinical Practice

The nurse educator in clinical practice interweaves the practice role as a professional nurse with the teaching role of an educator. Increased concerns over quality assurance emphasize continuing competency in the practice area. Also of concern for nursing faculty is maintaining competency in clinical skills.

The meaning of the role professional in any discipline has implications for a lifelong commitment to continuing education. Nursing faculty as professionals fulfill the role in academia (Gortner, 1984, p. 5). Because nursing is a practice discipline, the nurse educator must meet both academic and clinical commitments. Therefore, teaching theory and practice in nursing define the professional teaching role. Collaborative efforts by nursing educators and nursing service generate knowledge in the clinical area to enhance the curriculum (Jarratt, 1983, p. 501).

The professional practice role of the nurse educator may become an essential role for the nursing faculty. In some institutions of higher learning, clinical practice is a major part of the role of the nursing faculty (Spero, 1980, p. 24). One possibility is a faculty appointment that includes direct practice as a clinical specialist, a role for the nurse educator.

The implementation of the practice role of the professional nurse may vary according to the scope of the state's nursing practice act. Through the practice act of a specific state, the professional nurse is licensed to perform minimal practice expectations within the role as a registered nurse. State boards usually specify the educational requirements for teaching nursing. The nurse educator bases the teaching role on the legal practice of nursing, but teaching students at the baccalaureate level goes beyond the minimal mandated state requirements.

Any expansion of the practice role is controlled through the mandated practice acts. Extended roles of nurses and roles of clinical specialists and nurse practitioners are mandated in many states. Roles vary as to activities considered part of the role (Bigbee, 1984, p. 110). Nursing faculty who teach these roles to graduate students have the responsibility of knowing the parameters of the practice act. Inherent in the role, faculty practice is maintaining competency for practice and continuing education.

The clinical nurse specialist role is often not practiced by the nursing faculty due to time constraints or policy conflicts. Some nurse educators are not prepared as clinical nurse specialists. Some faculty maintain the intellectual, interpersonal, and technical skills to practice as clinical specialists on weekends and summers when not employed at the college. The role and the competencies needed by the clinical specialist are the subject of a study by Wyers, Grove, and Pastornio (1985, p. 207).

Almost always, the teaching role of the nursing faculty member encompasses a specific nursing specialty. The teaching assignment is usually performed within that specialty. Ideally, the nurse educator teaches in the area of practice. The preparation for role as faculty in nursing requires the maintenance of clinical skills.

How the nursing faculty member remains competent to practice and to teach what is currently practiced is a challenge. Learning how the nurse educator meets the demands for the time necessary to practice within the faculty role is important. The nurse educator is already overburdened with time and energy commitments and is reluctant to add practice to the role (Dickens, 1983, p. 121). What is certain is that nursing faculty in the college system must demonstrate excellence in teaching, research, and service to the community (McCarthy, 1981, p. 163).

In 1984, Holt (p. 448) stated: "It is practice that should serve to generate new knowledge, validate theory in practice and generate research." Practice is an excellent source for scholarly publication (Langford, 1983, p. 517). Faculty practice allows nurse educators to serve as role models for students and to provide clients with a high quality of care. Nurse educators who have managed to balance their time among the various roles of practice experience greater job satisfaction (Nichols, 1985, p. 90). In some settings, a pattern is established that considers teaching as practice.

Maintaining expertise in the clinical area, improving the quality of care, and generating economic resources for the nursing program are rationales offered by the proponents of faculty practice. Direct financial compensation to the faculty performing the practice has been suggested (Holm, 1981, p. 657). The nurse educator who practices role is identified as one who accepts the responsibility for the development of the nursing profession (Langford, 1983, p. 517).

The clinical practice of the faculty is a debatable issue in nursing education.

Practice is proposed for some faculty as a criterion of tenure. Whether faculty practice enhances the role of the nurse educator is a suggested subject for research (Wakefield-Fisher, 1983, p. 210).

The amount of faculty practice and whether it should occur while the nurse educator is teaching students or when the students are not present remains a question. Nevertheless, clinical practice in some dimensions is in transition. It could evolve into one of the major role tasks of the nurse educator. But the time for practice must be shared with the time for the five other major role tasks. In addition, many related role tasks exist that are student and faculty related.

RELATED ROLES

Student-related Roles

Recruiter. Student recruitment has become a vital function of long-term academic program management. An effective marketing strategy greatly influences recruiting efforts (Grabowski, 1981). College administrators have been evaluating the cost per student for the recruiting process (Dressel, 1978, p. 137).

Some college nursing programs employ full-time or part-time recruiters. For the faculty, recruitment is a major task. A selective admission model in nursing programs is utilized in many colleges. However, employment trends, available resources, and the number of students may predict the future admission models based more on successful recruiting efforts.

Although recruiting was not a traditionally accepted role in academia for the nurse educator, now it is. In the 1980s, nursing education programs have experienced the results of decreasing numbers of high school student graduations, declining college enrollments, escalating educational costs, and decreasing governmental support (Ford, 1982). Also, the increasing numbers of more attractive careers for women claim the available students. Student recruiting in the college system is a potential major task.

The role of recruiting for the nurse educator encompasses many interrelated activities with some overlapping into advisement. Articulation of the prerequisites to the program, requirements for admission, the curriculum itself, and the financial aid available should be anticipated by the faculty involved in recruiting. Genuine interest, receptivity, and motivation have further described the qualities of the nurse educator in the recruiting role. More effective faculty recruitment has taken place when the faculty has been committed to the process of recruitment (Buckley, 1980, p. 50).

An example of the scope of the nursing faculty role in recruiting is the recruitment of the newer adult learner into the baccalaureate program for registered nurses. Also, students who were college graduates with no previous nursing are enrolled. Curricula are developed with marketing efforts focused on the needs of future students.

Master's and doctoral students are more easily recruited for flexible and individualized programs. Programs that are perceived by potential students as meaningful to personal and professional development are desirable. Some doctoral programs are suggested exclusively as the future preparation for scholarly professional nursing practitioners and nursing investigators (Lutz & Schlotfeldt, 1985, p. 143). The marketing plan for a program dictates many of the recruiting activities necessary for a full enrollment of students.

An analysis of the nurse educator's role in recruiting activities is necessary. Once defined, recruiting expectations and workload standards for the faculty can be identified. The measurement of recruiting efforts by nursing faculty is becoming more important. Recruiting, however, is a related task for the nurse educator but one with increasing priority.

Advocate. Since the early 1970s, patient advocacy has been an established role for professional nursing (Fay, 1978). The concept of advocacy was extended to students by the development of the Bill of Rights for Students of Nursing (National Student Nurse Association, 1975). *Advocacy* is defined as the act of defending or pleading the case of another. The basic role of an advocate is to inform and to support the decision of another, abide by it, and defend the right of the individual to make the decision.

For nursing faculty, the role of the advocate is viewed as complex and with many risks. The general knowledge requirements for the advocate role include many categories: information, support, systems analysis, social ethics, complex medical issues, social laws, and politics. An adequate knowledge base on professional education and professional practice is also required (Kohnke, 1982, p. 315).

Applying the concept of advocacy, the nursing faculty treats the student with regard and respect. The faculty represents the student's cause or best interests in matters pertaining to the student and some aspect of the learning situation. The role of student advocate carries great responsibility.

The stress of collegiate education is no different for nursing students and, indeed, may be more stressful. The faculty in nursing are able to offer much guidance to students. The faculty advocate assists the student to analyze self, needs, and interest patterns. Advocates help to prepare students to make decisions that are more compatible to the student as an individual (Knefelkamp, 1980, p. 15).

As with other advocacy roles, the nursing faculty give professional information, assistance, or an opinion to the student, but the student makes the decision for action (Curtin, 1983). The nurse educator's role as an advocate is teaching the student how to make responsible decisions and how to accept a poor decision once made and convert it into a profitable learning experience for the future.

Preceptor. Supervision preceptors have been in existence since early days and are used in professional nursing education in a variety of forms. Although use of preceptorates is a form of teaching, it is a variation of the traditional teaching model.

The requirements for the preceptor are usually a graduate degree in nursing and experience if accreditation criteria are met. Supervisory arrangements for clinical preceptors are one of the related role tasks of the nurse educator. When preceptors are used, settings for clinical experiences have been increased. More opportunities for students are available for hands-on experiences. Clinical preceptorates were established for the newly employed graduate nurse. The new nurses were assigned to preceptors for the first six months to a year of their initial employment. The preceptor acted as a role model and guided the experiences of the new nurse (McGrath & Koewing, 1978, p. 12).

Other models involve the nursing faculty as the preceptor. The faculty preceptor model is used for primary nurse care practitioner students. This model requires the faculty member to be an experienced educator and a nurse practitioner (Helmuth & Guberski, 1980, p. 39).

The more contemporary model for preceptors involves the nurse educator as a faculty facilitator and the agency nurse as the preceptor. In some situations, the agency nurse in the preceptor role is more a resource person and less a supervisor or instructor (Henneman, 1983, p. 98). The role of the nurse faculty with preceptors is to arrange for each student assignment with a nurse preceptor. The preceptor needs continuing supervision, administrative support, and guidance from the faculty throughout the course. Clearly written role descriptions and evaluation tools are necessary for the preceptor and the student (Limon, Bargagliotti, & Spencer, 1981, p. 433).

Usually the student is assigned to the preceptor to learn hands-on skills and procedures. Some consideration is given to compatible matching between students and preceptors. The nurse educator who carefully selects the preceptor, the student, and the site is more often able to facilitate a positive learning experience.

The site may offer unusual services and resources to clients, enriching the opportunities for the student. The preceptor shares specialized knowledge and skills with students that are unique not only to the site when the nursing instructor is present, but also when only the preceptor is present. The learning experiences are based on the objectives of the course and the individualized goals and objectives of the student (Bergeron, 1983, pp. 89–95). The periodic monitoring of the learning experience by the nursing faculty during the course is necessary. All three, student, preceptor and faculty, participate in the evaluation. All three may evaluate the student's performance.

When faculty arrange a preceptor experience, the continued learning of both the student and the preceptor is possible. Preceptors add an innovative dimension to nursing education. Establishing a preceptor for students is a challenging related role task for the nurse educator.

Tutor. The role of the nurse educator as tutor is limited and difficult to differentiate from advising and counseling (Marks-Maran & Procter, 1983, p. 72). Tutoring involves academic assistance given to the student outside the classroom. The additional assistance is individualized and personalized instruction given at the student's pace. In nursing education, tutoring has been perceived as either an unstructured helping function or a structured "tutorial course" of instruction. Reviewing, remembering, and practicing difficult content under the direction of another person has been considered tutoring by Stephenson (1984, p. 283).

Some tutoring is delegated by the assigned nursing faculty to other faculty and to students who are known to have mastered the content in question. Students with weaknesses utilize tutoring for courses within the nursing curriculum and in other nonnursing courses. Nursing students often need tutoring in mathematics and science courses.

Tutoring is considered a form of coaching for nursing educators. It is advantageous to anticipate the student's need for tutoring (Smoyak, 1978, p. 361). Tutoring is an important related role task for the nursing faculty.

Faculty-related Roles

Administrative Governance. Administrative governance is the process of decision making towards determining the goals of institutions of higher learning. The process involves students, faculty, administration, and trustees. The shared governance approach has been effectively used in other academic programs prior to being utilized in nursing (Porter-O'Grady & Finnigan, 1984). Colleges employ faculty governance for consensual participative decision making (Rice & Bishoprick, 1971, p. 97). In 1981 (Ozimek, 1981), governance was found to be one of the four rights of the faculty, in addition to economic security, equitable workload, and working conditions.

Governance is the opportunity of the faculty to make decisions and to affect change in the decisions made by others. Decisions and policy formation are made through the interactions of the nursing faculty group and the college administration involved in governance (Rustia, 1983a, p. 68). Consensus is usually achieved through committee structures that use democratic methods.

Committees are micro-subsystems of the faculty. Departments and programs operate for the most part through committees. Faculty interactions with the college system take place through another group of committees. The committee unit performs the work of governance for the faculty. Most work is done through a system of formal committees. Faculty choose committees, or are elected by peers or appointed for committee membership. The successful operation of a faculty organization depends to a great extent on the effectiveness of the committee units, provided the committees operate with an updated set of bylaws.

Committees are both standing and ad hoc. The types of committees in the college system have included the committees of personnel, admissions, research, curriculum, faculty development, library, student grievance, bylaws, and others (Andruskiw, 1983). The types of committees in the clinical setting on which the nurse educator may serve would include audit, safety, in-service education, or standards. In the community setting, the nurse educator is invited to serve as a consultant—member on a committee—for example, quality assurance, education, planning, or fiscal committees.

Nurse educators serve on boards in the community, contributing expertise to long-range planning, evaluation, and goal setting. In return, faculty gain valuable experience and recognition (Chapman, 1983, p. 176; Robb, 1981, p. 27). Sometimes, nursing faculty serve in a less formal group for a specific purpose, i.e., interest, task force, action group, work group, interdisciplinary group, and community group.

The role of an effective committee member involves participative attendance on a regular basis and being willing to function as chairman and share the secretarial duties. A nurse faculty member serves on two to five committees, depending on the size of the department. Committees are vital mechanisms for helping nurse educators explore ideas, interact with others, and help peers (Andruskiw, 1983, p. 39). These groups can form a foundation that later may develop as a peer support group.

Participation in academic governance requires immeasurable amounts of time and energy. Committee work consumes the time of many members (Redman & Barley, 1978, p. 31). When people are allowed to participate in decision making within an organization, however, morale is enhanced. Productivity is also increased in major faculty tasks (Kelley, 1978, p. 17).

Areas of governance were studied by Bahrawy (1985, p. 89). A majority of nursing faculty agreed that participation in governance is limited by lack of socialization into the faculty role as well as heavy teaching and clinical assignments. Further, frequent absences from campus due to nursing-related activities, time required for professional practice, increased clinical loads because of retrenchment, and centralization of authority during financial exigencies are other activities that hinder faculty participation in governance.

Faculty, in this study, sometimes agreed that participation in governance was difficult for women faculty in the male-dominated professoriate. However, governance is supported by the faculty members' belief in governance and in collegiality. Faculty believe that participation increases morale and productivity, and governance is effective when supported by the nursing dean and the tenured faculty (Bahrawy, 1985).

The rewards of active involvement in governance for the nurse faculty are realized through the faculty awards, merit, tenure, and promotion. For this reason, governance activities have a higher priority than other related roles for the nurse educator.

Professional Organization Member. A faculty-related role but one of significant importance in nursing involves membership in professional nursing organizations. Organizations are necessary for solving the problems and facing the issues of the nursing profession as a unified group. Entry into practice, credentialing, and the appropriate educational system for nurses are some examples of professional problems. The public questions why the memberships in the nursing organizations are not greater. Nonmembership is considered a lack of professional identity (Lewis, 1978, p. 323).

Types of organizations for nurse educators include the American Association of Colleges of Nursing, Commissions and Councils of the American Nurses' Association, the National League for Nursing, and Sigma Theta Tau. Sections of organizations encouraged for nurse educators include the specialty and subspecialty nursing organizations, i.e., Occupational Health Nurses Association and Critical Care Nurses Association. Organizations with disease-focused groups include the American Cancer Society and the American Heart Association. Nationally, the American Public Health Association and the American Association for Higher Education are multidisciplinary for many different health care professionals and educators.

While membership in an organization involves various levels of participation, many educators of nursing are members. Regular attendance at meetings and conferences or serving on a committee as member or chairperson is desirable. Becoming an officer or a member of the board is a rewarding faculty task (Kibrick, 1981).

As a member of a profession, nurses who are faculty members are expected to participate in the activities of professional organizations (Van Ort, 1985, p. 27). Organizations need support and to represent the total population. When functioning as a unified group, problem solving on issues of concern to the total professional group is more effective. Nursing organizations can present a strong and autonomous position for the profession.

A market survey (Dommel & Rauen, 1985, p. 272) asked nurse members of the state organization of the National League for Nursing if the services provided were what the members wanted. Services of value were the newsletter, earning continuing education units, and reduced rates on publications and programs. Other positive comments regarded the promotion of quality home care and community health nursing in their state. The services needed included quarterly membership meetings with an educational focus and more frequent general meetings. When nursing faculty actively represent an organization they have an opportunity to pursue preferred services.

The policy statements adopted by leading nursing organizations have supported change in health care services patterns. Nurse educators have participated in these actions (Moore & Oakley, 1983, p. 504). A few hours of time for regular monthly meetings can be integrated into the total role of the faculty. The benefits resulting from the participation in organizations will gain both personal and professional satisfaction. Benefits are derived from getting to know others and networking. Word-of-mouth employment opportunities also exist.

Education Provider–Consumer. The related role of education provider–consumer is one that describes a dual role for the faculty member, providing continuing education for others or being oneself a consumer of continuing education.

Providing for professional and educational growth in others includes planning, organizing and conducting courses, seminars, colloquia, workshops, symposia, conferences, and all types of in-service education. Nursing education for others requires the identification of learning needs, assessment of the learners, mastery of learning and teaching theories, motivation, time, and mastery of the content to be taught (Puetz, 1981). Faculty who are continuing education providers can offer peer-reviewed quality programs for credit.

Continuing education is of the highest quality to meet accreditation standards. Content of substantial nature, pre-tests and post-tests, and a certificate awarding a specific number of continuing education units at the completion are offered (Kelly, 1981b, p. 64). A conceptual framework should exist for continuing education curricula, according to Wise (1980, p. 320).

Although not totally accepted, mandated continuing education for nurses exists in several states. The nurse educator in the college setting is one responsible for planning programs to assist nurses in the community to meet this requirement (Wasch, 1980, p. 119).

In order to promote and market continuing "lifelong learning" education programs for nurses, nursing faculty assess the participant and the motivation of the participant. Motives of participants include desire for professional knowledge, improvement in social welfare skills, professional advancement, acquisition of credentials, compliance with authority, relief from routine, and improvement in social relations (O'Connor, 1980, p. 260). Continuing professional growth is measured through earning continuing education units or CEUs, academic credit, or participation in credit-free learning opportunities.

Continuing education for faculty is necessary for several reasons. Maintaining current knowledge and skills for a specialization in an area of professional nursing in which one teaches is the most important. Earning credits toward the terminal degree is necessary for faculty on tenure-track appointments. Professional role enhancement is also a reason (i.e., stress and time management test construction, statistics, research, writing, computer skills, and capability with audiovisual equipment).

Faculty development is another term for professional growth, and the philosophy of faculty development varies from college to college. A philosophy of faculty development is a set of beliefs about how nursing faculty should be prepared, what they should be doing, and how they should be rewarded. It included beliefs about measuring and assuring continued growth (Hart, 1982).

Faculty development is described as collective or individual. Individual faculty should set goals and development plans that span 5 years and are evaluated periodically. Goal setting is a part of faculty evaluation. Priorities for activities in the plan may change from year to year, but the 5-year goal should not. All faculty development activities are the responsibility of the individual nurse educator (Abruzzese, 1984). Career-oriented personal and professional growth are motivating factors.

In a study in 1981 (Lane et al., 1981, pp. 115–116), the barriers to faculty development were found to be personal and institutional in nature. Among the personal barriers noted were finances, lack of interest or necessary child care, home management responsibilities, and social responsibilities. Institutional barriers were workload, faculty scheduling, lack of release time, and insufficient financing.

The extensive professional commitments of the faculty ranked continuing education as a low priority. As providers or consumers of continuing education, nurse faculty benefit from the experiences. Either providing or participating in continuing education or earning degree credit adds to the scholarly activities necessary to demonstrate for retention, tenure, or promotion in the academic system.

Political Leader. The related role of the nurse educator as a political leader is a full-time responsibility in itself. Political awareness and action by nurse leaders are imperative as legislation impacts on the health care delivery system (Davis, 1982). Active nursing faculty are more likely to influence the profession through political, economic, and social activities. Political socialization integrated throughout the curriculum better prepares students for political leadership. Some vital decisions on health care should involve nurses and politicians (Archer, 1982, pp. 109-147).

Most policymakers have limited knowledge about the role of nursing. A primary responsibility for the nurse educator as a political leader is to be knowledgeable about the political process. Nurse faculty who are articulate influence decisions on legislation for patient care, nursing education, and nursing research. To be a credible resource person for information about current legislation affecting patient care and nursing education is the goal of the nurse educator in this role (Stein, 1982, p. 302).

Faculty in nursing can seek out leadership activities as a means to develop positive relationships with those in politics. This should be encouraged. Encouraging other faculty to register to vote, writing thank-you letters to legislators for support of nursing bills, attending and participating in district community meetings, or sponsoring a fund raising event are other activities that are encouraged (Maraldo, 1982, p. 1104). Political leadership can be further demonstrated by nurse educators who can volunteer for policy-making activities. Serving on community boards and task forces are examples (Smith, 1983, p. 135).

A survey measuring nurses' political activities revealed agreement that participation in politics is compatible with nurses' professional roles. The larger percentages of nurses participated in voting for president, mayor, and city council and registering to vote (Moore & Oakley, 1983, p. 505).

Political subjects that were reviewed in the nursing literature between 1976 and 1982 include politics, power, organizational power, civic lessons, education of the legislative process, Washington politics, lobbying, how-to-subjects, political strategies, legislative issues, and regulatory issues (Lake & Lamper-Linden, 1983, p. 334). The articles provide valuable background information for nurse faculty who plan a more active role in politics.

Assertiveness is considered a prerequisite for the politically active faculty. The skill of the nurse educator in a political role is an ability to assert nursing's case. Volunteer campaign work for both candidates and initiatives, participation in the activities of the political parties, and political action committees were the strategies suggested by Archer (1984, p. 114).

Other strategies for nurse educators involve participation on legislative task forces and establishing nursing legislative subcommittees (Rowell & Knauss, 1981; Underly, Doxsey, & Reeves, 1981). Networking with other nurses and non-nurses who have similar political interests is an effective strategy. Nurse educators who become political role models strengthen nursing's position. Nurse educators who are politically united for action can influence professional and health care issues (Baker & Hart, 1981).

Involved and committed nurse educators have demonstrated the power to influence politicians and other nurses (Rothberg, 1985). Nurse educators are among the professional nursing leaders with the responsibility to exercise power and influence peers.

Mentor. Nurse educators teach others directly or indirectly through being role models. Faculty assist peers through the mentoring process. The mentoring process is effective in developing educational leaders in nursing.

SUMMARY

With the constraints on time and energy, the nurse educator is confronted with several major and related role tasks. How time for tasks is prioritized and how energy for tasks is expended in pursuit of the multiple roles remains the challenge to be met in the search for the rewards.

REFERENCES

Abruzzese, R. S. (1984). Continuing education needs of faculty. *Dean's Notes, 53*. Pitman, N.J.: Anthony J. Jannetti, Inc.

Andruskiw, O. (1983). A socio-humanistic model of administration. In M. Conway & O. Andruskiw (Eds.), *Administrative theory and practice: Issues in higher education in nursing* (pp. 15–16, 38–49). E. Norwalk, Conn.: Appleton-Century-Crofts.

Archer, S. E. (1982). Political strategies for nurses' involvement. In S. E. Archer & P. A. Goehner (Eds.), *Nurses: A political force* (pp. 109–147). Monterey, Calif.: Wadsworth Health Science Division.

Bahrawy, A. (1985). Faculty participation in academic governance of baccalaureate programs in nursing: Summary. *Proceedings and Abstracts* (p. 89). 3rd Annual Meeting, Research in Nursing Education, Society for Research in Education, San Francisco.

Baird, S. C., Biegel, A., Bopp, A., Dolphin, N. W., Ernst, N., Hagaedorn, M., Malkiewicz, J., Payton, R. J., & Sawatzky, G. (1985). Defining scholarly activity in nursing education. *Journal of Nursing Education, 24,* 143–147.

Baker, N. C., & Hart, C. A. (1981). Nurses in action. *Nursing & Health Care, 11,* 130–132, 168–169.

Bergeron, C. T. (1983). What precepting is. In S. Stuart-Siddall & J. M. Haberlin (Eds.), *Preceptorships in nursing education* (pp. 89–95). Rockville, Md.: Aspen Systems Corporation.

Bigbee, J. L. (1984). Territoriality and prescriptive authority for nurse practitioners. *Nursing & Health Care, 5,* 106–110.

Bolton, J. G. (1984). Educating professional nurses for clinical practice. *Nursing & Health Care, 5,* 385–389.

Bossenmaier, M. (1979). Students evaluate academic advising. *Nursing Outlook, 27,* 787–791.

Brown, J. S., Tanner, C. A., & Padrick, K. P. (1984). Nursing's search for scientific knowledge. *Nursing Research, 33*(1), 26–32.

Buckley, J. (1980). Faculty commitment to recruitment and retention of black students. *Nursing Outlook, 28*(1), 46–50.

Chapman, J. J. (1983). Serving on the board of directors of a nonprofit organization. *American Journal of Maternal Child Nursing, 8,* 173–176.

Charron, S. A. (1985). Role issues and the nurse educator. *Journal of Nursing Education, 24*(2), 77–79.

Conrad, C., & Pratt, A. (1983). Making decisions about the curriculum. *Journal of Higher Education, 54*(1), 16–30.

Curtin, L. (1983). The nurse as patient advocate: A commentary. *Dean's Notes, 4*(5). Pitman, N.J.: Anthony J. Jannetti, Inc.

Davis, C. K. (1982). Nurses' decade of political power? *Briefly Noted, 2*(4), Viewpoint #13.

Dickens, M. (1983). Faculty practice and social support. *Nursing Leadership, 6,* 121–127.

Diers, D. (1983). Editorial: Clinical scholarship. *Image: The Journal of Clinical Scholarship, 15*(1), 3.

Dill, D. D. (1982). The structure of academic profession: Toward a definition of ethical issues. *Journal of Higher Education, 53,* 255–267.

Dixon, B. (1977). Defining the role of instructor. In *Instructional innovations: Ideals, issues, impediments* (pp. 58–64). New York: National League for Nursing.

Dommel, D., & Rauen, K. (1985). Keying in on members' needs. *Nursing & Health Care, 6,* 273–274.

Dressel, P. L. (1978). *Handbook of academic evaluation* (pp. 137, 359–366). San Francisco: Jossey-Bass Publishers.

Dressel, P. L., & Mayhew, L. (1974). *Higher education as a field of study* (p. 332). San Francisco: Jossey-Bass Publishers.

Eble, K. E. (1973). *Professors as teachers* (p. 170). San Francisco: Jossey-Bass Publishers.

Fagin, C., & McGivern, D. (1983). The dean and faculty development. In M. Conway & O. Andruskiw (Eds.), *Administrative theory and practice: Issues in higher education in nursing* (p. 212). E. Norwalk, Conn.: Appleton-Century-Crofts.

Fawcett, J. (1984). The metaparadigm of nursing: Present status and future refinements. *Image: The Journal of Nursing Scholarship, 16,* 84–87.

Fay, P. (1978). Sounding board: In support of patient advocacy as a nursing role. *Nursing Outlook, 26,* 252.

Ford, L. (1982). The golden rule. *Briefly Noted, 2*(3), Viewpoint #9.

Gortner, S. (1984). Knowledge in a practice discipline: Philosophy and pragmatics. In C. Williams (Ed.), *Nursing research and policy formation: The case of prospective payment* (pp. 5–16). New York: American Academy of Nursing.

Grabowski, S. (1981). *Marketing in higher education* (ERIC Research Report No. 5). Washington, D.C.: American Association of Higher Education.

Hart, S. (1982). A proposed philosophy of faculty development. *Briefly Noted, 2*(2), Miscellaneous #6.

Heckenberger, N. (1983). The future in master's and doctoral education in nursing. In *Perspectives in nursing 1983–85* (pp. 179–185). New York: National League for Nursing.

Heidgerken, L. (1965). *Teaching and learning in schools of nursing* (p. 33). Philadelphia: J. B. Lippincott.

Helmuth, M. R., & Guberski, T. D. (1980). Preparation for preceptor role. *Nursing Outlook, 28*(1), 36–39.

Henneman, J. (1983). The needs of a new preceptor. In S. Stuart-Siddell & J. M. Haberlin (Eds.), *Preceptorships in nursing education* (pp. 97–101). Rockville, Md.: Aspen Systems Corporation.

Hollshwandnen, C. H., Kinsey, D., & Paradowski, M. B. (1984). Teacher-practitioner-researcher. *Nursing & Health Care, 5*, 144–149.

Holm, K. (1981). Faculty practice: Noble intentions gone awry? *Nursing Outlook, 29*, 655–657.

Holt, F. M. (1984). Theoretical model for clinical specialist practice. *Nursing & Health Care, 5*, 445–449.

Jarratt, V. (1983). "The time has come," the Walrus said, "to talk of many things". *Nursing and Health Care, 4*, 498–503.

Jones, J. J. (1983). University liability in program advisement. *Nursing & Health Care, 4*, 83–84.

Kelley, J. (1978). Factors affecting decision making in academic nursing from the viewpoint of faculty. In *Decision making within the academic environment* (pp. 13–22). New York: National League for Nursing.

Kelly, L. Y. (1981a). *Dimensions of professional nursing* (4th ed.) (p. 298). New York: Macmillan.

Kelly, L. Y. (1981b). Continuing education: Step two. *Nursing Outlook, 29*, 64.

Kibrick, A. K. (1981). Accountability, review boards and the lay participant. *Nursing & Health Care, 11*, 124–129.

Knefelkamp, L. (1980). Faculty and student development in the 80's: Renewing the community of scholars. *Current Issues in Higher Education, 5*, 13–24.

Kohnke, M. F. (1982). Advocacy: What is it? *Nursing & Health Care, 3*, 314–315.

Lake, R. S., & Lamper-Linden, C. (1983). A subject bibliography on legislative and political action. *Nursing & Health Care, 4*, 334–337.

Lancaster, J. (1984). Bonding of nursing practice and education through research. *Nursing & Health Care, 5*, 379–387.

Lane, E. B., Lagodna, G. E., Brooks, B. R., Long, N. J., Parsons, M. A., Fox, M. R., & Strickland, O. L. (1981). Faculty development activities. *Nursing Outlook, 29*, 112–118.

Langford, T. L. (1983). Faculty could practice if—and other myths. *Nursing & Health Care, 4*, 515–517.

Lawrence, S. A., & Lawrence, R. M. (1983). Curriculum development: Philosophy, objectives and conceptual framework. *Nursing Outlook, 31*, 160–163.

Lewis, E. P. (1979). The professionally uncommitted. *Nursing Outlook, 27*, 323.

Limon, S., Bargagliotti, L. A., & Spencer, J. B. (1981). Who precepts the preceptor? *Nursing & Health Care, 11*, 433–436.

Loomis, M., & Krone, K. (1980). Collaborative research development. *Journal of Nursing Administration, 10*(12), 32–35.

Lutz, E., & Schlotfeldt, R. (1985). Pioneering a new approach to professional education. *Nursing Outlook, 33*, 139–143.

Maraldo, P. (1982). Politics: A very human matter. *American Journal of Nursing, 82*, 1104–1105.

Marks-Maran, D., & Procter, P. (1983). Hello Tutor—goodbye? *Nursing Times, 79*(33), 72.

Mayhew, L. (1970). The undergraduate student: Needs and problems. In M. Hardee, *Faculty advising in colleges and universities* (p. 1). Washington, D.C.: American Personnel Guidance Association.

McCarthy, P. A. (1981). Will faculty practice make perfect? *Nursing Outlook, 29*, 163.

McGrath, B. & Koewing, J. (1978). A clinical preceptorship for new graduate nurses. *Journal of Nursing Administration, 8*(3), 12–18.

Moore, E., & Oakley, D. (1983). Nurses, political participation and attitudes towards reforms in the health care delivery system. *Nursing & Health Care, 4*, 504–507.

National Student Nurse Association (1975). Student Bill of Rights. *Imprint, 22,* 49–50, 67–68.
Nichols, C. (1985). Something for everyone. *Nursing Outlook, 33,* 85–90.
O'Connor, A. B. (1980). The continuing nurse learner: Who and why. *Nurse Educator, 5*(5), 24–27.
Ozimek, D. (1981). Rights and responsibilities of students and faculty. *The Dean's List, 3*(2).
Pinkava, B. K., & Haviland, C. P. (1984). Teaching, writing and thinking. *Nursing Outlook, 32,* 270–272.
Porter-O'Grady, T., & Finnigan, S. A. (1984). *Shared governance for nursing: A creative approach to professional accountability.* Gaithersburg, Md.: Aspen Systems Corporation.
Puetz, B. E. (1981). *Continuing education for nurses.* Gaithersburg, Md.: Aspen Systems Corporation.
Redman, B. K., & Barley, Z. A. (1978). On the governance system of university of schools of nursing. *Journal of Nursing Education, 17*(7), 27–31.
Reed, S. (1983). Educational mobility: From concept to reality. In *Perspectives in nursing 1983–85* (pp. 157–165). New York: National League for Nurses.
Rice, G. H., & Bishoprick, D. W. (1971). *Conceptual models of organizations* (pp. 1–97). E. Norwalk, Conn.: Appleton-Century-Crofts.
Robb, S. S. (1981). Nurse involvement in institutional review boards: The service setting perspective. *Nursing Research, 30*(1), 27–31.
Rothberg, J. S. (1985). The growth of political action in nursing. *Nursing Outlook, 33,* 133–135.
Rowell, P. A., & Knauss, P. J. (1981). The legislative task force: A method to increase nurses' political involvement. *Nursing Outlook, 29,* 715–716.
Rustia, J. (1983a). The relationship between university missions, relevant professional practice and policy formation: An illustration. *Nursing & Health Care, 4,* 66–71.
Schroeder, D. (1981, November). Learning needs of the new graduate entering hospital nursing. *Nurse Educator,* 10–17.
Schurr, G. M. (1982). Towards a code of ethics for academics. *Journal of Higher Education, 53,* 318–334.
Schweer, J. (1968). *Creative teaching in clinical nursing* (pp. 1–39). St. Louis: C. V. Mosby Co.
Scriven, M. (1982). Professional ethics. *Journal of Higher Education, 53,* 307–317.
Smith, E. D. (1983). Nurses in policymaking and volunteerism. *Nursing & Health Care, 4,* 135–137.
Smoyak, S. A. (1978). Teaching as coaching. *Nursing Outlook, 24,* 361–363.
Spero, J. (1980). Nursing: A professional practice discipline in academia. *Nursing & Health Care, 1,* 22–25.
Stein, K. Z. (1982). Grassroots political action: Organizing a legislator's day. *Nursing & Health Care, 3,* 302–304.
Stephenson, P. (1984). Aspects of the tutor-student nurse relationship. *Journal of Advanced Nursing, 9,* 283–290.
Stevens, B. J. (1985). Does the 1985 nursing education proposal make economic sense? *Nursing Outlook, 33,* 124–127.
Sullivan, E., & Brye, C. (1983). Nursing's future: Use of the Delphi Technique for curriculum planning. *Journal of Nursing Education, 22,* 187–189.
Trombley, T. B., & Holmes, D. (1980). The changing roles and priorities of academic advising. *Current Issues in Higher Education, 2*(1), 20–24.

Underly, N., Doxsey, K., & Reeves, D. M. (1981). Establishing a nursing legislation subcommittee. *Nursing Outlook, 29,* 717–719.

Van Ort, S. R. (1985). *Teaching in collegiate schools of nursing.* Boston: Little, Brown.

Vemulapalli, G. K. (1984). The unnecessary conflict between teaching and research. *The Chronicle of Higher Education, 28*(22), 64.

Wakefield-Fisher, M. (1983). The issue: Faculty practice. *Journal of Nursing Education, 22,* 207–210.

Wasch, S. (1980). The role of baccalaureate faculty in continuing education. *Nursing Outlook, 28,* 116–119.

Weiss, S. (1984). Educating the nursing profession for role transition. *Journal of Nursing Education, 23*(1), 9–14.

Wise, P. Y. (1980). Curriculum development in continuing education: Option or necessity? *Nursing Outlook, 28,* 318–320.

Wyers, M. A., Grove, S. K., Pastorino, C. (1985). Clinical nurse specialist: In search of the right role. *Nursing & Health Care,* 203–307.

3

Teaching and Service

Alice LeVeille Gaul, Ph.D., R.N.

The teaching of a practice discipline such as nursing presents unique problems as well as rewards to the nurse educator. A brief look at the history of nursing education will assist the new nurse educator to understand some of the current challenges. Schools of nursing proliferated in the first quarter of this century, with the number growing from 423 to over 2000 (Christy, 1980). There were not adequate instructors of nursing available to accommodate this growth, and in some cases, there were none. The result of the unavailability of faculty to accommodate the increasing student population was that student nurses were taught by other nurses and by senior students. The students were essentially responsible for the functioning of the hospital, and in reality, there was little or no formal education.

Eventually, hospitals began to hire registered nurses to function as head nurses, and one component of that role was to assume the teaching responsibility for the student nurses. The main thrust of nursing education at this point was still the acquisition of nursing skills to be acquired on the hospital wards. As late as 1942, the National League for Nursing described the faculty of a school of nursing as composed of clinical nursing supervisors and head nurses, as well as the usual academic components of a faculty (Christy, 1980).

In the 1950s, education monies were moved out of practice settings and into schools of nursing, which resulted in the employment of full-time faculty not connected with the service setting. This move, while defining and strengthening the educational foundations of nursing, also allowed persons with little or no actual nursing experience to become teachers of nursing solely by virtue of earned academic degrees. The greater the distance of the faculty person from service, the greater the possibility that the knowledge, both experiential and acquired, required for the effective teaching of the discipline of nursing will not be available to the educator.

The nurse educator, due to the nature of the profession, must be both an expert educator and an expert clinician. The new teacher of nursing must enter the discipline doubly prepared and is required to learn, to experience, and to conquer the challenges of both classroom and clinical teaching. This challenge is compounded by the fact that the two different types of teaching require different methodologies, different evaluation strategies, and at times, two different personalities in the same individual. The reward of teaching in a practice discipline is the continual enhancement of both individual and professional growth in those striving to achieve excellence as nurse educators.

DEFINING THE INSTITUTION'S EXPECTATION OF TEACHING

The logical point at which to begin exploring expectations of the novice nurse educator is at the beginning. Underlying that sage advice is the assumption that one knows where the beginning is. The beginning in nursing education is and always must be the curriculum. In order to define the institution's expectations, the educator must become familiar with the philosophy of the school, the goals of the school and of its sponsoring organization, the conceptual framework of the curriculum, the integrating strands of the curriculum, and the organization of the curriculum. Knowledge of these will logically lead the teacher to the course-specific objectives relevant to his or her assignment. Such material will probably have been provided prior to the interview or upon appointment. If it was not, the individual should request it immediately. This material provides valuable insights as to not only what content must be taught, but how it should be taught, how the student is to be regarded in the teaching–learning situation, and evaluation methodologies.

The new teacher can be assured that inherent in faculty expectations is adherence to the existing curriculum model and philosophy of the faculty, which must provide the framework, not only for evaluation of the curriculum itself, but for all who teach within it. A new teacher, in accepting the faculty appointment, has agreed to abide by the existing curriculum framework and philosophy and can expect to be evaluated by it.

In addition to the conceptual issue just discussed, some of the more pragmatic ways to determine institutional expectations follow. Most institutions will provide the new teacher with some sort of faculty handbook that clearly outlines the privileges and expectations of the faculty role. In addition, most colleges of nursing have some sort of policy manual outlining the specific evaluation policies for faculty. Identify the mechanisms for evaluation of classroom and clinical training as well as the criteria. Obtain copies of all standard evaluation forms, which will clearly identify criteria. Do not assume that faculty evaluation is automatic. Many schools expect faculty to make their own arrangements for evaluation.

The faculty role also consists of service to the college and to the parent institution if appropriate. Find out from the faculty handbook, an immediate supervisor, or a trustworthy colleague the committee service expectations of a new faculty member. If not appointed to a committee, volunteer for one that is of interest. This is an excellent way to learn more about the institution, the curriculum, and new colleagues.

The military service has a phrase "command performance" to denote functions for which invitations are issued, but attendance is mandatory. The same concept exists in faculty life, and it behooves the new teacher to determine which meeting and school functions are "command performances." This information should be provided in new faculty orientation, but if it is not, make an effort to obtain it either from a supervisor or a colleague, for it is, in fact, one of the faculty expectations.

Underlying the ancillary roles of faculty is the clear expectation that the first and foremost role of the nurse educator is that of an expert teacher. The definition of that term, however, remains elusive. Some of the qualities possessed by an expert teacher must include: knowledge of the subject that is current; an ability to present that knowledge in a clear, cohesive manner; the ingenuity to tailor the presentation of that knowledge to the learning styles and needs of both the students and the course content; the ability to recognize cognitive dissonance within the students and to either utilize it in the teaching–learning process or to correct it; and a clear comprehension that teaching–learning is a mutually interactive process requiring alertness and flexibility on the part of the teacher if the goal of learning is to be accomplished. A limited unpublished survey done by this author to determine the characteristics of a teacher most valued by students in a particular university setting revealed that 87 percent of the respondents valued "enthusiasm of the teacher for the content" over such qualities as "well prepared," "cites current literature," and "paced the course appropriately." The second most valued quality was "respected the students as individuals." The qualities given to the students to rate were those listed on the university-required student evaluation of faculty teaching.

Ford (1983) has identified from the literature and from personal experience characteristics, which excellent teachers exemplify. They are: commitment to the profession, as manifested in scholarly activities such as research and publications and in increasing growth in knowledge of subject content; the ability to communicate ideas in a direct, concise fashion so that they can be clearly understood by students; expertise in decision making, open-mindedness to new experiences, and the ability to rationally process information; involvement and expertise in advisement and counseling along with the ability to sustain the interpersonal relationships with students that underlie this role; the ability to grow in the profession and to learn and utilize techniques that improve teaching year to year; the ability to organize and to present information to students as well as to offer guidance to students for individual growth and development; the ability to view each student as an individual without prejudice; and the ability to consistently present quality material with sufficient depth and breadth.

DEFINING THE TEACHER'S EXPECTATION OF TEACHING

Nurses enter the field of nursing education for a variety of reasons, but generally underlying them is the belief that the educator can effect change in the profession. Kramer (1974) proposed that nurses who could no longer tolerate the ambiguity of the bureaucratic setting chose, as one alternative to service, nursing education. The underlying drive that causes a nurse to seek the necessary higher degrees and a position in nursing education should be clearly identified by the individual, for the key to both the rewards and the frustrations of nursing education lies in the underlying motivation of the individual.

The beginning teacher should clearly identify, in a realistic manner, both self-expectations and expectation of the position prior to assuming its responsibilities. Of the two, self-expectations frequently tend to be the most unrealistic. One cannot assume a new position composed of a multitude of roles, comprehend it, and perform it perfectly within the first week. To expect that is unrealistic and will ultimately lead to frustration and a possible loss of self-esteem. It is important to understand that this is not generally the institution's expectation of a new, inexperienced faculty member. More appropriately, the new educator will set both short-term and long-term personal goals related to understanding of the curriculum, class preparation, and performance of the faculty role; prioritize them; and then begin to accomplish them one by one. Personal goals, like learning goals, must be measurable and realistic. Long-term goals should reflect utlimate career goals, but be measurable at intervals, such as at 1, 3, and 5 years. This will allow the new educator to begin immediately to share in the rewards of the educator's role, which are more often measured day to day by small accomplishments such as a student's grasping a difficult concept than by major changes in either the attitude or performance of the profession.

SELECTING A LEARNING THEORY

During the educational experience of the new teacher, no doubt a substantial amount of time was spent in the study of the different learning theories. It is appropriate that all available theories be closely examined and studied at that time. Prior to actually beginning teaching, the new educator should closely examine personal beliefs regarding the teaching–learning experience and select the theory or theories most congruent with those beliefs in order to provide a framework for an individual approach to the educational experience. The individual's beliefs should, of course, not be in conflict with the beliefs of the faculty and the sponsoring institution as set forth in the philosophy.

Some educators prefer an eclectic approach to the theory base underlying their personal teaching–learning philosophy because of the belief that there is an advantage to be gained in terms of potential depth and variability of less structure. While the selection of a theoretical approach to education is highly personal, the eclectic approach for the educator has inherent dangers in that it might not provide the needed structure and guidance for one forging unfamiliar territory.

A new educator with an eclectic theoretical approach may find that when a dilemma is presented, there is no organized systematic set of inter-related concepts to provide guidance, but rather a series of concepts that present conflicting guides to the resolution of the dilemma. Another inherent danger in selecting pieces and parts of many learning theories is that the concepts selected may not have the same meaning when viewed separately from their theoretical base. Therefore, they do not provide the educator with the necessary sound theoretical framework from which to view and to shape the teaching–learning experience from both the perspective of the student and of the educator.

The type of program and the age of the learner will also dictate the type of theoretical approach that is necessary. Educators must have a vital interest in the selection and development of theories of learning, since curriculum development revolves around the selection of learning goals and the methods of achieving them (Conley, 1973). Everything a teacher does is guided by the theory he or she subscribes to. For example, an educator who views the learner as self-motivated will not generally utilize "pop quizzes" to assess the student's ability to complete the reading assignments. The teacher bases daily decisions on a systematic body of theoretical knowledge; without it, there would be no cohesiveness and no evidence of a long-range rational purpose or plan (Bigge, 1976).

This is not to imply, however, that the same theory will be equally useful in all situations. The well-prepared educator will have a knowledge of the major learning theories and be able to select one appropriate to the learning situation. Pragmatically, however, the educator generally selects one that he or she is most comfortable with to guide the personal approach to the teaching–learning experience. It is not within the scope of this chapter to present a compendium of the various learning theories, but the reader is referred to the many books available on this subject, and should, indeed, have one in his or her personal library.

MENTORSHIP

The nurse educator receives academic preparation in a variety of programs, which prepare their graduates at the master's and doctoral level. On the graduate, just as on the undergraduate level, the programs are varied and diverse. It is possible to obtain a graduate degree in nursing with little or no formal course work and no practical experience in educational content. Teaching in and of itself is a practice discipline. It is not enough to be able to speak to it, to read about it, and to write about it. If one is going to be successful, one must also be able to do it. If there was no opportunity to have a guided practicum in the classroom as a portion of graduate education, the first actual teaching experience will begin with the appointment in a school of nursing. When not provided with formal opportunities, how then does the new educator get the necessary guidance, feedback, and direction for growth that a novice requires? One answer is to find an experienced teacher who will become a mentor.

A *mentor* by dictionary definition is "a wise and trusted counselor or teacher" (Morris, 1969, p. 820). The concept of mentorship has existed for centuries in other disciplines and is based upon a Greek mythological character named Mentor who was Odysseus' trusted counselor (Morris, 1969). Mentorship, in nursing education, encompasses both the concept of counselor and of teacher. It is not a relationship, which can be assigned, but rather one that is selective in nature and one, which must be nurtured and allowed to develop at its own pace. The rewards in terms of personal and professional growth for both the mentor and the person being mentored are enormous, one of them being that eventually that distinction blurs. The relationship is so much more than simply the relationship of teacher, preceptor, advisor, or role model. It is a combination of all of these and has more subtle nuances difficult to describe. It is a relationship to be cherished and one that in its true form is still relatively rare in nursing.

How does one find a mentor? Since the relationship obviously does not materialize out of thin air and cannot be assigned, the new educator needs to begin to search for one. Since the mentoring relationship requires compatible personalities, one of the first steps must be to get acquainted with colleagues. Select some whose knowledge and teaching ability are particularly admired. This may or may not be the person who was assigned to you for orientation or one who teaches in the same area of specialization. Begin to go to these faculty members for assistance, feedback, and guidance. Gradually, the process of natural selection will take over and instinctive selection will occur. When ready, initiate a discussion of the mentoring relationship desired in order to determine if both parties want to agree to pursue it. Then begin to nurture and to develop it. It is important to emphasize that this discussion has centered around the concept of mentorship in the classic sense and is not to be mistaken for or to replace the concept of a person who orients and advises new faculty.

STRUCTURING TEACHING TO THE CURRICULUM

The relationship between the curriculum, the institutional expectations of teaching, and the evaluation of nurse educators has been addressed. The type of curriculum will also guide the content and in many cases the methodology appropriate for presenting it. Peterson (1983, pp. 93–94) has identified several trends in nursing curricula:

- Movement away from blocked curricula to ones with integration of content around broad themes or threads
- General progression away from the medical system model to a conceptual, nursing-care-process model
- Development of curricula based upon conceptual models. More recent developments are beginning to include emphasis on better curriculum, including the emphasis on testing frameworks used by faculty and students
- Increased emphasis, particularly in baccalaureate and graduate curricula, on the research process and use of research findings in planning care
- Inclusion of themes such as standards of care, care planning, and quality assurance within undergraduate professional curricula
- Derivation of curricula from a detailed framework of goals and objectives
- Implementation of the academic model of the laboratory in the clinical component of the curriculum

- Increased use of the techniques and strategies of individualized and independent instruction

With curriculum ever changing in response to societal needs and trends, as well as the evolution of nursing knowledge, the educator must be constantly vigilant that teaching does in fact reflect the curriculum. It is an old saying that teachers tend to teach as they were taught. A nurse educator oriented to the medical model specialty approach may have substantial difficulty adjusting to a more conceptual framework, such as nursing process, in presenting content. That is not to imply that it cannot be done, but every nurse educator, experienced and inexperienced alike, must be ever vigilant and examine closely from the framework of the individual curriculum what and how he or she is teaching. If each educator is allowed to present content in the manner and from the framework that he or she prefers, the result is likely to be students who have bits and pieces of nursing knowledge but no organizational framework from which to view and integrate a cohesive body of professional knowledge.

As curricula were being integrated in response to the evolving conceptual theoretical approach to nursing education, different teaching methodologies were formulated in an attempt to respond to the needs of this approach. One of these was team teaching, the concept of which was to utilize specialty knowledge of faculty to organize and present content, in an interactive format, with the theoretical or conceptual framework as the unifying theme. The implementation of team teaching, when it worked, was effective and satisfying to both the faculty and the students. However, in many instances, it did not work because educators had difficulty adjusting their presentations to this new format. What resulted was "turn teaching" with each member of the teaching team presenting content from the framework of the traditional medical model, in turn and with little more than lip service to the organizing theoretical or conceptual framework. The students were left with successive lectures representing different medical-model specialty content, no perception of an organizing framework, and substantial difficulty in integrating the content into a body of knowledge useful to them.

Another inherent danger of not structuring teaching exclusively within the curriculum model is that of overloading students with content. It is another old adage about teachers that they tend to teach *all* that they were taught. Without the control of curriculum structure, the educational experiences of the educators will tend not only to become integrated within the content, which is in the most part desirable, but become content in and of itself, which is not. Addition of content to existing courses rarely results in deletion of other content to make room for it, but rather the overloading of a course. The system of checks and balances that exists within a curriculum should prevent the addition of new content without the agreement of the curriculum committee and the faculty. However, this system only works when the educator desiring to add the content presents it to the appropriate channels for inclusion in the curriculum. The educator who, in a burst of enthusiasm for content newly learned, decides to add it independently to the course, bypasses the system of curriculum checks and balances and ultimately may jeopardize the students' learning of essential content.

TEACHING IN THE CLASSROOM

Preparing for the first classroom experience is often fraught with feelings of anxiety and terrible self-doubt. The imposter syndrome or the belief that "now surely someone will discover that I don't belong here" frequently surfaces. These very natural feelings are often compounded by the fact that the professional college teacher was never formally trained for the job. "Most university teachers are turned loose on their students without any formal recognition that teaching is an art that requires its own knowledge and skill" (Schwartz, 1980, p. 236). Other authors stress the belief that one learns by doing, that given an underlying educational foundation within the discipline all that there is to teaching can be learned by teaching (Hutchins, 1936). That notion, while true at least to some degree, tends to be very circular and may be construed to imply that unless one has taught for a period of time, one cannot be an excellent teacher. There are inherent qualities associated with excellence in teaching that the new nurse educator by virtue of personal characteristics and education brings immediately to the discipline. Chief among these are knowledge and love of nursing and a deep respect for the learner as a valued human being. Education must be understood in terms of the human interaction between teacher and student because the development of the learner as a person rests on the impact of one human being upon another (Buber, 1955). Armed with these two most important qualities of an excellent teacher, the new educator is certainly well prepared to begin teaching.

SELECTION OF A METHODOLOGY

Armed with the specific learning objectives and an understanding of their articulation within the curriculum and the organizing framework, the teacher must select a methodology to present the content. The objectives in and of themselves as well as the class size will guide the methodology. Two of the most preferred strategies are presented.

Lecture

The lecture, although disparaged by many, continues to thrive as a teaching methodology and remains both a popular and a valid means of presenting content. In order to be effective, the lecturer must have a clear understanding of both the purpose and the structure of the lecture. The purpose of the lecture is to achieve one or more of the following objectives: to transmit information, to create interest, and to promote understanding (Woods, 1983). The structure of the lecture is closely allied to its purpose and can be categorized as the classical model, the problem-centered model, and the sequential model.

The classical model has its criterion as its main theme, and information is grouped around that unifying theme. This model is best suited for the transmission of information. The problem-centered approach utilizes a particular identified problem as the focus of the presentation, and information is presented in the form of arguments and hypotheses as possible solutions. The problem-centered approach is most suited to creating interest. The sequential model consists of a series of linked statements building and leading toward a possible conclusion. This approach is most suited to promoting understanding (Woods, 1983).

In a lecture whose purpose it is to transmit knowledge, understanding cannot be expected to occur immediately, but will occur later when the learner has had time to analyze and to reflect upon the knowledge presented. For example, if content is presented relative to the use of arterial blood gases in determining the acid-base status of patients, the initial purpose is to transmit information, which can later be assimilated through reinforcement by analysis and synthesis. The purpose of the initial lecture is to present the content in as clear and concise a manner as possible, to present the organizing framework for comprehension, to clarify the concepts, and to aid the student in determining the relationships between them.

A given lecture may not be limited to one purpose and, in fact, may incorporate all of them. Therefore, it is incumbent upon the lecturer to be very clear when preparing the lecture as to the purpose of each segment and to utilize effective strategies for each. It would be ludicrous to begin a presentation of the content on interpretation of arterial blood gases with a series of clinical case studies that require the students to determine the acid-base status of the patient from the laboratory values and the clinical signs and symptoms. Yet that particular learning activity within the framework of a sequential lecture format would be very appropriate after the information was presented and when the purpose is to promote understanding of the content.

The formal presentation of ethics content in nursing curricula is a current challenge to nurse educators. Few schools of nursing have separate ethics courses, and this very essential content, in the majority of curricula, must be integrated throughout the existing courses (Beardslee, 1983). Inferred from this is that while that ethics content may be best taught in a seminar discussion format, the majority of nursing students will have it presented to them in a lecture format. An example of selecting the appropriate purpose and structure of the lecture is presented using ethical content as an example.

Example: The Ethics Lecture. The first purpose of the proposed ethics lecture is to stimulate interest in the subject. The lecturer must be aware when preparing that the degree of interest of the lecturer in the subject and the students' desire to learn the content may not be and are often not necessarily congruent. This is often true when the content deviates from the students' perception of content that is essential to "real nursing" practice. It would not be necessary to stimulate students' interest in interpretation of arterial blood gases since it is likely that they will perceive that as a necessary conceptual skill. The need for understanding of and the ability to use ethical theories in resolving ethical dilemmas will, in all likelihood, take some selling. Hence, the first purpose of the ethics lecture must be to create interest, while the first purpose of the acid-base lecture would be to present information. Using a problem-centered format, the lecturer may present some of the common ethical dilemmas experienced in nursing practice, and present many of the possible and often conflicting solutions with all the ramifications to the nurses involved, such as loss of employment, role conception, and conflict with the existing authoritative structure.

The information portion of the lecture, best presented in the classical manner, would consist of the presentation of the major ethical theories concepts, as well as some decision-making model that allows for incorporation of these into the decision-making process. Finally, the portion of the lecture that provides for understanding of the content would utilize the sequential method of structuring content. In this example, that might be a presentation of an ethical dilemma with a step-by-step demonstration of the application of the major ethical theories to the ethical decision-making process. The end decisions would then be compared and contrasted and conclusions drawn. The amount of time available for presentation of the ethics content would vary from one period to many, depending on the curriculum.

Lecture Anxiety. Probably there is no situation that the new nurse educator finds more frightening than the formal lecture. This feeling is often compounded by watching new colleagues lecture with great poise and apparent ease. King (1973), in a study of university teachers' anxieties, found that the problem most raised by academicians is the anxiety they feel about the formal lecturing situation. Underlying this anxiety are feelings of self-doubt and often unrealistic self-expectations. For this reason, comfort in the lecture situation cannot be taught through methods or process. Each educator must deal with the individual's underlying feelings. Certainly success eases the self-doubts, thereby relieving some of the anxiety. Another very helpful method of dealing with lecture anxiety is the utilization of a relaxation technique. By keeping the physical self in a state of relaxation and the mind focused, one can concentrate on the job at hand, the lecture, rather than personal anxieties. An internal pep talk is also very useful. After all, would you even be there if your dean or chairperson did not feel you were eminently qualified to serve as a role model for the novices in your profession and are clearly qualified to present the content at hand?

Lecture–Discussion

Instructional discussion creates a learning situation that is focused upon the application of knowledge rather than acquisition of facts. This method employs carefully planned questions that allow students to develop skills in thinking and problem solving (Gaut & Blainey, 1982). One of the main advantages to this teaching strategy is that it demands participation and preparation from all participants, who must formulate ideas and opinions, defend opinions, and draw conclusions. It requires intensive preparation by the teacher if it is to be effective. The role of the teacher is not "to go with the flow" but to carefully pose questions and guide the discussion.

Some of the inherent problems in the lecture–discussion methodology that require teacher intervention are generating the discussion, dealing with nonparticipants, and handling arguments. It is most disconcerting, when you have prepared for a lecture–discussion format, to enter the room armed with pertinent questions, pose the starting point of the discussion, and look about at a group of ten blank faces. It is important for the teacher to create a milieu conducive to this format. The students must know each other and must feel safe in expressing their opinions. Some type of "getting-to-know-you" exercise is appropriate on the first class day and until a comfortable, nonthreatening atmosphere exists. It is important for the teacher to realize that the students may already know one another very well, and may, in fact, have some history of conflict. The specific points of conflict between the group members need not necessarily be resolved, but the teacher must create an atmosphere in that class that renders them nonpertinent to the present situation. Nonparticipants need to be drawn out to participate in the discussion in a nonthreatening manner. This may be accomplished by capitalizing on nonverbal cues, by nonthreatening direct questions, or by asking the nonparticipant to assist another student in the reasoning process about a specific question. When the students feel safe and are committed to their opinions, it is possible that arguments may result. If the teacher retains control, arguments can be very stimulating to the discussion, but if the teacher loses control, they can be very destructive, not only to the class, but to the entire course. Salient points of each side of the argument should be summarized, and then the participants and the entire class should be guided through the steps of conflict resolution while being assisted to distinguish between facts, emotions, and opinions.

Another role of the teacher in lecture–discussion is to summarize the discussion at the appropriate time so that there will be closure on one point and the group is free to move on. There are no specific pre-established points at which summarization is necessary. However, if summarization occurs too early, discussion will be terminated, resulting in frustration to the group. If it occurs too late, the group may very well have lost focus and direction. Typically, when there are no new points being made or when the same points are being stated, it is time to consider closure through summarization. This author believes that closure is not necessary at the conclusion of each class period. If the discussion is unfinished, summarizing it to conform with the constraints of classroom time may result in premature closure and the inability to renew the discussion. The cognitive dissonance generated by an unfinished discussion may very well cause the students to continue to creatively think about the issue in the intervening time between class periods and to return to class ready to pose innovative solutions.

The limitations of the lecture–discussion method include group size and objectives to be covered. Because of the nature of the group process necessary in this format, the group size is ideally 10 or fewer and not over 15. Due to financial constraints existing in most colleges of nursing, class size usually exceeds this number in most courses. The objectives to be covered must be higher-level cognitive objectives such as application, analysis, and synthesis. This is not an appropriate format for presentation of new material. This strategy can be very difficult for the new educator, who may be uncertain of the ability to control and guide the discussion. It is, however, an exciting method of teaching that not only results in accomplishing the learning objectives, but also conveys to the students the notion that they are professionals whose ideas and opinions are valued and respected. As with other strategies, the novice nurse educator should attempt it when appropriate, rejoice in the successes, and forgive and learn by the errors.

STUDENT EVALUATION

Student evaluation methodology or testing presents challenges to the nurse educator. The subject is highly complex and requires knowledge of test and measurement best discussed in books and courses dealing with that subject. Therefore, this discussion will center around the logistics of testing rather than the content of constructing and evaluating testing.

Planning the chronological placement of tests requires consideration of the objectives covered both in terms of cognitive level and number. Another very pragmatic consideration must be the amount of total classroom time the teacher wishes to devote to testing. Balancing these two factors along fairness to the students in terms of collecting adequate data with which to evaluate them is difficult. There can be no absolute guidelines as to number of tests, types of tests, or number of items on a test. The decision factor must be that all objectives are measured at the appropriate level and that information obtained from the testing is sufficient to evaluate the students' grasp of the concepts.

Similarly, the type of testing, such as multiple-choice, short-answer, or essay, is dictated by the objectives and by the teaching strategy. If one has used a lecture–discussion format through the course, the measurement of learning would be most appropriately through some type of discussion questions rather than multiple choice. If one has used predominantly the lecture format, than multiple-choice items are appropriate measuring devices.

Whatever the format, the items should be closely evaluated for both content and construct validity. If the new teacher decides to use items drawn from a test pool, it is still a responsibility to closely evaluate the items. It is very dangerous to assume that just because questions have been previously used in testing, they are valid either according to construct or content. Once the teacher uses them, they become that teacher's responsibility, regardless of who wrote them. Test blueprinting is a valuable means to assure objectives are covered and leveled according to the appropriate cognitive domain. However, the educator must realize that this is simply an aid in the construction and evaluation of tests. Blueprinting is not an end in itself, and when rigidly implemented, can contribute to a fractionalized view of nursing (Peterson, 1983).

Test anxiety, experienced by many students, presents unique problems to the educator. On one hand, they must evaluate the student by the objective data obtained by testing and, on the other, support the student in what can be construed as a crisis situation. The anxiety engendered by the testing situation can be manifested in varying degrees of anxiety, physiological symptoms, and even acute panic attacks. Obviously, if severe physical symptoms or acute panic attacks are present, the student needs immediate referral for professional counseling, as measurement of learning cannot occur in that situation. Less severe anxiety can interfere with the student's performance during testing. The educator should learn to recognize when this might be the underlying cause of poor student performance on tests so that the students may be referred for counseling and assistance with test-taking skills. Test-taking skills are certainly important for all students, but particularly for nursing students, who must ultimately take a 2-day test for professional licensure. Early recognition and intervention by the nurse educator of test-taking problems can ultimately result in success for the student in the licensure examination.

CLINICAL TEACHING

The teaching role of the nurse educator consists of classroom teaching and clinical teaching. Planning, structuring, and evaluating clinical teaching requires different strategies from those needed in the classroom. Clinical teaching is enormously consuming in terms of physical, cognitive, and emotional energy of the teacher as well as of time.

In general, the clinical laboratory hours are planned on a ratio of 1:2 or 1:3, that is, 3 hours of clock time for every 1 hour of credit. For example, a 3-credit-hour course is typically taught 3 hours a week over a 15-week semester. A 3-credit-hour clinical course utilizing a 1:3 ratio is taught 9 hours a week over a 15-week semester. Obviously, this has an impact on the load a nurse educator carries versus the teaching load carried by educators of other disciplines. Educational cost-effectiveness is, as in other businesses, eventually reduced to numbers. The nurse educator carrying a clinical course as well as theory courses will, on paper, look exactly like another educator carrying all theory courses because the bottom line is credit-hour generation by the teacher. Therefore, the extra clinical contact hours become irrelevant in terms of academic load because the credit-hour generation is still 3 hours. Historically, academic nursing has argued that because of the necessary clinical component, nursing faculty need more time, more money, less credit-hour generation, and less education than other academic faculty (Infante, 1981). This argument may be counterproductive to nursing as an academic discipline, and without doubt, in the current economic crisis facing not only academic institutions but society at large, it is becoming less and less credible. The beginning nurse educator is entering the discipline at a time when great changes are forthcoming in terms of clinical teaching, including increasing use of independent learning experiences and clinical preceptors. The exact role of clinical teaching needs to be redefined, objectives examined, and methods of accomplishing those objectives most economically in terms of education, time, and money evaluated.

Planning and Conducting the Clinical Experience

Clinical experiences, like all learning activities, are planned on the basis of the curricular objectives. The selection of a credit-hour to clock-hour ratio should be accomplished through careful examination of the type and the availability of the desired learning experiences. Clinical experience for the student should serve as the integrating catalyst for the knowledge acquired in the classroom. The educator must be very clear as to the exact objectives to be achieved through clinical experience. Many clinical experiences are conducted as if the objective is total clinical competence of the student. That is clearly unrealistic. If a faculty believes that learning is conceptual in nature and that learning allows for transfer of conceptual information into a behavioral situation, then that faculty is unjustified in planning, for example, for repetitive clinical performance of skills. Still the question remains: How much is enough? Clearly the ideal amount of clinical laboratory time is one of the most discussed but least scientifically studied issues of nursing education (Infante, 1981).

Clinical objectives must be clearly defined to the student as well as expectations of the behaviors necessary to accomplish them. If this is not done at the beginning of a clinical rotation, most of the students' energy will be consumed in trying to figure out just what the clinical teacher wants of them. When the students' energy is directed in this manner, they are not cognitively free to integrate knowledge in the manner necessary for learning to occur. If written work, such as nursing care plans, is to be required, the educator should carefully go over each component with the students. Clearly defining the expectations of the teacher also greatly reduces the students' anxiety over the clinical situation.

The method of patient assignment must be decided and presented to the student. There are equally convincing arguments for instructor selection versus student selection of patients. Ultimately, the decision rests in the level of the students' ability, the objectives to be accomplished, and the degree of responsibility the instructor wishes to give to the student. If the student is to select the patient, the criteria for selection must be made clear. A welcome trend in nursing education is toward independent learning experiences in the clinical laboratory. Depending on whether or not this is implemented, students are either given a set of clearly defined objectives or allowed to develop their own and assume responsibility for implementing them with the aid of either a clinical preceptor or an instructor. This places the responsibility for learning with the learner, where it should reside, and promotes a less paternalistic, more collegial educator–student relationship. The ultimate responsibility of the nurse educator in the clinical setting is to guide experiences and to evaluate learning; it is not to supervise. The learning that occurs in the clinical setting is highly individual and beyond the control of any teacher. The concept of guidance is the opposite of that of supervision and includes supporting, stimulating, and facilitating the actions of nursing students so that they can begin to gain a concept of themselves as qualified practitioners (Infante, 1981).

The clinical conference is generally considered an integral portion of the clinical experience. It provides an opportunity for the students to achieve integration of their experiences through the guidance of their classmates and instructor. It also increases the variety and depth of experiences through the mutual sharing by students of their experiences. It is similar in nature and requires many of the same skills as the lecture–discussion. Conference time is limited, very precious, and should be utilized wisely. To that end, the teacher should have specific objectives regarding what is to be accomplished during each conference. However, a great deal of flexibility is also necessary, since the clinical learning experiences are so situational. Often the objectives must be changed at the last minute in order to deal with the more acute needs of the students at the time. It is a travesty of the intent and benefit of clinical conference to use that time to present new content to the students. When this occurs, it is time for the faculty to closely examine the curriculum to determine where that content ought to be lodged.

Clinical Evaluation

Evaluation of the students' clinical performance must be based upon the specified learning objectives. The process of evaluation should be clearly outlined to the students at the beginning of the clinical experience. The assignment of a clinical grade is frequently fraught with uncertainty, because while objective data may have been meticulously collected, there is still a substantial element of subjectivity involved. It is clearly impossible to see all behaviors demonstrated by a student during a clinical rotation, so the grade must be calculated on what is, hopefully, a representative sample of those behaviors. The assignment of letter grades to a clinical practicum requires that the clinical teacher not only evaluate specified behaviors, but categorize them in terms of A, B, C, D, and F behaviors. Pragmatically, the distinction between an A student, a C student, and an F student is generally clear. The distinction, however, tends to blur in the case of the B and the D student. Nonetheless, the B and D grades must be as amenable to justification as the others. Many institutions, for that and other reasons, have turned to a strictly pass/fail grading system. This method improves clinical evaluation because it requires only the differentiation between two levels of competence (Fowler, 1983). A study done by Hayter (1973) investigated letter grading by 31 clinical instructors based upon films of students in three clinical situations. The inter-rater reliability was extremely poor. For example, in one situation using the same student example, the educators marked 1 A, 10 Bs, 16 Cs, 3 Ds, and 1 F.

Whatever the grading system in use, the nurse educator needs to ensure that adequate data are available to justify the grade. This present some difficulties because a strictly evaluative climate is not conducive to the self-directed learning that is to be accomplished in the clinical setting. It is likely that if the student perceives that every teacher–student interaction is being recorded as data for evaluation, the guidance of the instructor will not be sought. Clarify to the students just when they are to be evaluated and what is to be evaluated. One useful method is to inform them that because of patient safety and legal implications, they will be evaluated constantly on the critical (safe versus unsafe) behaviors. However, the rest of the evaluation process will be based upon progression of behaviors that are measured by achievement of the objectives for the experience. This should relieve the students of the expectation that any behavior must be performed perfectly the first time and reinforce the notion that nursing is a profession that accepts and rewards growth.

The preferred method of collecting and compiling data is anecdotal notes. The student has the right to see the anecdotal notes kept regarding their performance at any time. Therefore, the language and content of these notes should be carefully selected. Describe the facts of the behavior, using only who, what, when, how, and where. Do not draw conclusions, assess blame, or make a value judgment. To do so leaves one open to legal action. The purpose of the anecdotal notes is to document the validity of grades, which includes passing as well as failing grades.

SERVICE

As previously identified, another component of the role of nurse educator is that of service. Service to the college and the sponsoring institution is generally construed to be participation in the work of the various committees. Service to the community is generally construed to be activities within the professional organizations and the sharing, without renumeration, of professional expertise with the community. The underlying concept of service is that the nurse educator is a leader in the profession and as such has a civic responsibility to the institution, which employs him or her, and to the community, professional and otherwise, in which he or she resides.

Service to the College

Committee work within a college of nursing provides a variety of opportunities for personal and professional growth. The selection of committees in which to participate can provide the new educator opportunities for understanding the curriculum and the power structure (formal and informal) of the college, as well as promoting collegial relationships. The power committee in any college is the curriculum committee. While it is unlikely that a new faculty member will be asked to join that committee, there are usually opportunities for participation in various ad hoc and subcommittees convened by the curriculum committee. If those opportunities are not available, the new faculty person is well advised to attend some of the meetings as an observer.

Some of the other committees, which may be beneficial to the person adjusting to the role of new faculty, are the bylaws, social affairs, research, and library committees. The degree of participation in committee work should be commensurate with the individual's goals.

Service to the Community

Membership and active participation in professional organizations is a clearly defined expectation of faculty in schools of nursing. Membership in the American Nurses' Association is generally required, and membership in the National League for Nursing and appropriate specialty organizations is strongly recommended. If there is a chapter of the International Honor Society for Nursing, Sigma Theta Tau, in the area, membership in that is also encouraged. The degree to which one participates in the activities of these organizations is governed by constraints of time and energy. It is clearly evident that intense involvement in all of the organizations along with the expectations of teaching, scholarship, and personal life is impossible for most people. One solution is to become involved in the activities of the organization, which can contribute to your personal career goals. As your goals evolve or are met, change the focus of involvement. This approach is mutually beneficial to both the organization, which obtains an active committee worker, and to the faculty, who provides for opportunities to meet personal goals through service.

The sharing, as part of a civic commitment, of professional skills to the community is extremely rewarding. By doing this, the nurse educator is often able to accomplish both personal and professional goals as well as engender a sense of belonging and pride. Some examples of community service might include participation in American Heart Association programs and service on various boards and committees such as the Mental Health Mental Retardation Board or the research committees of various hospitals. Planned presentations and workshops to both professional and nonprofessional groups are interesting and can be very rewarding.

An example that epitomizes the concept of community and professional service is that of a nurse educator who, after having done a longitudinal epidemiological study of rape in a metropolitan area, utilized the results of that study to develop a presentation on rape prevention, which was delivered to PTAs, women's organizations, schools, police departments, and other organizations. That same nurse educator was instrumental in the planning, development, and implementation of a rape crisis center. The educator benefited, the university benefited, and the community was richer for this individual's professional commitment.

There may be some tendency for the burdened faculty person to view the service obligation as one more brick added to the load that a nurse faculty member is expected to carry. However, faculty overload is not something that can be weighed in pounds. Perhaps it is best weighed in terms of benefits to the individual, to the profession, to the organization, and to the community. The last three are clearly evident; the first may take some examination. The obligations of teaching, service, and scholarship are not to be viewed as mutually exclusive activities that take place within a vacuum. They should be interactive processes, with participation in one benefiting the other, and when viewed that way, the faculty expectations become more desirable. For example, the nurse educator who is regarded as a clinical expert and invited to give workshops or classes in a hospital setting has gained phenomenal credibility with the nursing staff, which will ultimately benefit the clinical students. The nurse educator who speaks to community groups is always recruiting, not only for the college but for the profession of nursing. Service on boards and committees as well as speaking engagements often result in identification of researchable problems and easier access to populations as well as material for publications. The obligation for service to the college and to the community is an integral portion of the role of professional educator and should be viewed as a privilege.

REFERENCES

Beardslee, N. Q. (1983). *Survey of teaching ethics in nursing programs and the investigation of the relationship between the extent of ethics content and moral reasoning levels.* Unpublished doctoral dissertation. Greeley, Colo.: University of Northern Colorado.

Bigge, M. L. (1976). *Learning theories for teachers* (3rd ed.). New York: Harper & Row.
Buber, M. (1955). *I and thou* (Walter Kaufman, Trans.). New York: Charles Scribner's Sons.
Christy, T. E. (1980). Clinical practice as a function of nursing education: An historical analysis. *Nursing Outlook, 28*(8), 493–497.
Conley, V. C. (1973). *Curriculum and instruction in nursing.* Boston: Little, Brown.
Ford, M. L. (1983). Excellence in teaching: What does it really mean? *Improving College and University Teaching, 31*(3), 137–141.
Fowler, G. A. (1983). Guidelines for clinical evaluation. *Journal of Nursing Education, 22*(9), 402–404.
Gaut, D. A., & Blainey, C. G. (1982). The lecture approach to teaching nursing—method or habit? *Nursing and Health Care,* February, 73–77, 82–84.
Hayter, J. (1973). An approach to laboratory evaluation. *The Journal of Nursing Education, 12,* 17–22.
Hutchins, R. M. (1936). *The higher learning in America.* New Haven: Yale University Press.
Infante, M. S. (1981). Toward effective and efficient use of the clinical laboratory. *Nurse Educator,* January–February, 16–19.
King, M. (1973). The anxieties of university teachers. *Universities Quarterly, 28,* 69–83.
Kramer, M. (1974). *Reality shock: Why nurses leave nursing.* St. Louis: C. V. Mosby.
Morris, W. (Ed.). (1969). *The American Heritage dictionary of the English language* (p. 820). Boston: American Heritage Publishing Company and Houghton Mifflin Company.
Peterson, C. J. (1983). *The nursing profession: A time to speak.* New York: McGraw-Hill, 91–99.
Schwartz, W. (1980). Education in the classroom. *The Journal of Higher Education,* May–June, *51.*
Woods, J. D. (1983). Lecturing: Linking purpose and organization. *Improving College and University Teaching, 31*(2), 61–64.

4

Practice, Education, and Research

Gail C. Davis, Ed.D., R.N.

EVOLUTION OF COLLABORATIVE ROLES IN NURSING

"Collaboration," "bonding," "unification," "manpower sharing," and "partnership" are all terms, which have been used to describe the expanding role of the nurse educator. These terms have appeared in the nursing literature with increasing frequency since the 1960s. They describe the professional role, regardless of the place of employment, as one, which includes education, practice, research, and consultation (Christman, 1979a). The major focus has been on combining the practice and research dimensions with educational responsibilities. There are numerous kinds of arrangements, which support this type of professional role. The term "collaborative" will be the one used here to refer to these various types of arrangements. The discussion of the nurse educator's research and practice roles will be organized within the framework of the full professional role, since this is the ultimate goal of collaboration.

The practice dimension of nursing has always been strong; it is nursing's raison d'être. Research, on the other hand, has not generally been viewed by nurses as essential to this practice. Nurses have been slow in accepting research as a vital part of their role. Interestingly enough, the combination of these evolutionary aspects within nursing's development have led to the current "collaborative era." The present era is focusing on the return of nursing to its "roots" while, at the same time, nurturing and expanding these roots.

When nursing education moved from the hospital to institutions of higher education, e.g., colleges and universities, there was a perceived need to draw clear lines of distinction between practice and education. Initially, this may have been an essential part of the process of developing a necessary degree of autonomy for nursing education. A part of this evolution, though, was the loss of good role models as educators focused on the academic portion of their role and as the schism between practice and education grew. Nursing's evolution has now proceeded to the point of more objectively seeing the need for blending the best elements of both areas into the whole of nursing.

Research in nursing is evolving as part of the whole. Since research content is primarily considered to be graduate-level content, this portion of the role has emerged as an important one only as the profession has had more nurses prepared at the master's and doctoral levels. Initially, many of the studies conducted by nurses dealt with education and nurse-oriented problems, rather than clinical ones. Again, these studies reflected nursing's evolution. Only now is the profession at the point of seriously promoting clinically oriented research. This clinical orientation is supported by the collaborative approach, for the researcher "in a clinical setting is particularly constrained to do research which is very directly and visibly related to either the improvement of patient care or the minimization of costs for the care" (Larson, 1981, p. 75). Collaboration in research calls for the best efforts of all; it is described as "merging for the research process the talents of health care workers with a diversity of backgrounds and motivations" (Hinshaw, Chance, & Atwood, 1981, p. 33).

There are a number of reasons for supporting service–education collaboration, but the major one is to move the profession of nursing forward. This is the approach, which should lead to the development of a true professional nursing practice model based on research. That will take the best combined efforts of nurses working in all areas. MacPhail (1983, pp. 641–642) notes five reasons for collaboration and unification between nursing education and nursing service: (1) "to provide the best quality of nursing care," (2) "to provide an exemplary learning climate for nursing students and staff," (3) to promote "the development of nursing research," (4) to "resolve problems of nurse supply and demand," and (5) to promote the "interdependence of a school of nursing and organized nursing services utilized for students' practice and research." All are interrelated and point to the importance of improving the whole of nursing through the continuing development of nurses, nursing students, climate for service and education, nursing theory, and nursing curricula.

Early discussions of collaborative–unification models appeared in the literature in the 1960s; these appeared with increasing frequency during the 1970s and into the 1980s (Christman, 1979b; Hicks & Westphal, 1977; Powers, 1976; Schlotfeldt & MacPhail, 1969; Smith, 1965; Sovie, 1981a; Sovie, 1981b). The early approaches (University of Florida, Case Western Reserve University, University of Rochester, and Rush-Presbyterian–St. Luke's Medical Center) focused on organizational methods, which would support unification. By 1980, several models were available for those interested in implementing joint education–service ventures, and the need for this was well documented. The decade of the 1980s refocused the discussions of need. The added dimension was a greater emphasis on finances. The advent of the prospective payment system (PPS) under Medicare, along with a society, which was becoming increasingly aware of health care costs and more concerned with cost-effectiveness in health care, further emphasized the need for practice and education to work together to discover new approaches to the provision of nursing care. Now the first goal, as stated above by MacPhail, might be expanded: "to provide the best quality of nursing care in a cost-effective manner." This trend has also brought with it an impetus for clearly identifying the role and scope of nursing practice, as serious discussions between nurses and administrators of health care agencies take place about charging for nursing services.

CURRENT TRENDS

The American Association of Colleges of Nursing (Redman, Cassells, & Jackson, 1985) recently conducted the Generic Baccalaureate Nursing Data Project, which compiled and analyzed data provided by over 200 baccalaureate nursing education programs. Findings addressed the areas of faculty involvement in practice and research. Not quite half of the schools (47 percent) calculate research–scholarship time into the workload formula for faculty; this calculation of credit occurred with greater frequency in academic health centers and universities, as opposed to 4-year colleges. Collaborative arrangements between faculty and clinical facilities existed in a variety of forms. Those that were cited by more than half of the schools responding were: (1) research involving clinical nursing studies, (2) cosponsorship of professional nursing continuing education programs, and (3) adjunct professorship arrangements with clinical agencies (p. 375). The percentage of faculty holding joint or shared appointments with clinical agencies was 28 percent (p. 374).

The collaborative model may take a variety of approaches, both in terms of the kinds of functions, which might be included, and in the type of administrative arrangement. While there may be a number of ways to handle the administrative arrangements, the two most common types of joint appointments are (1) associate and (2) shared. The associate appointment does not involve any exchange of money by the education and service agencies. The nurse keeps the major appointment in either the educational or service agency and simply provides services for the other agency. A shared appointment implies that both agencies—clinical and educational—share in the compensation of the nurse who is providing services for both (Staff, 1985).

When working out the initial arrangements for a collaborative appointment, both the nurse educator and the two agencies involved need to decide what functions are most desirable for all. Obviously, the nurse involved will have an interest in and the ability to carry out the functions desired by both agencies. Evaluating this "fit" provides the basis for negotiation. For example, one collaborative model described by Sovie (1981b) points out that every nurse in the organization, regardless of whether the primary appointment is education or service, "is involved in practice, education, and research" (p. 30). This particular model (University of Rochester) allows each faculty member clinician to negotiate for the amount of time, which will be spent in the areas of education, practice, and research.

CURRENT CONSIDERATIONS

Before negotiating a collaborative role, each individual nurse will want to weigh the advantages and disadvantages from a personal perspective. It is often said that working in a joint appointment is "like having two full-time jobs." Unfortunately, this may prove to be true. The burnout rate is high. For this reason, the nurse needs to set very clear personal and professional goals and then really attempt to use them as a guide. Setting these goals can be enhanced by drawing upon the experiences of others who have worked in similar situations.

The advantages of collaborative arrangements which have been documented are many. A summary of these include the following:

1. Faculty maintain clinical competence and gain increased clinical credibility.
2. Faculty become better role models for students.
3. The learning climate is improved for both students and staff.
4. Colleagueship of nurses grows, regardless of primary work orientation.
5. Nurse work satisfaction is increased because of the opportunity to function in the full professional role.
6. Holding staff privileges facilitates the teaching and research roles of the faculty member.
7. Opportunities for continued learning are enhanced.
8. Consumer awareness of the professional nursing role is increased.
9. Quality of nursing care is increased.
10. Awareness is increased among nurses about the different roles they assume; thus, there is greater consideration of one another.
11. The motivation to become involved in nursing research increases.
12. Research relevant to nursing practice increases.
13. Innovative approaches to nursing and nursing education increase.
14. Applications of research findings in clinical practice increase.

All of the advantages sound wonderful—and they can be. As with any situation, however, there are some disadvantages, which need to be weighed. Hopefully, an awareness of these can assist the nurse in avoiding them or, at least, controlling them.

The disadvantages, which have been generally identified include:

1. Balancing the demands of the service agency, the educational agency, and research commitments may seem to require superhuman strength and commitment.
2. Receiving the proper recognition and incentive to continue in the collaborative role from the employing agencies may be a problem.
3. The issue of priorities (patient care versus education) may emerge from time to time, especially on holidays, weekends, and when patient census is high or staffing is limited.

4. Faculty recruitment may be a problem, especially in situations where practice does not receive high priority in evaluations for tenure and promotion.
5. Working out the arrangements for a collaborative appointment requires much administrative creativeness and time; thus, the appropriate detail may not be given to making the arrangements workable ones.
6. The freedom and autonomy necessary for the nurse to study nursing and report findings is not always assured or protected by the policies of the clinical agency.

By all means, there is a definite challenge to administrators of both educational and clinical agencies to make these appointments workable. Flexibility is a key. The numerous methods, which have been tried to date demonstrate that there is *no one way* to implement a collaborative project; in fact, arrangements of individuals within the same agencies may vary. Actually the goals, which need to be integrated, are those of the agencies involved, the individual nurse, and—perhaps most of all—the profession of nursing.

The remainder of this discussion focuses on some of the aspects of collaboration, which deserve the attention and careful consideration of nursing, individual agencies and their administrators, and the individual nurse. The major areas of the total professional role—practice, education, research, and consultation—are used as an organizing framework. There is some overlapping of content, since these areas are, by nature, integrated.

PRACTICE

Background

Practice is the essence of nursing. Any definition of nursing focuses on direct interaction with the patient or client. This began with Florence Nightingale's definition when she stated that nursing puts "the patient in the best condition for nature to act upon him" (Nightingale, 1884, p. 133). Henderson (1966, p. 15) later elaborated upon this:

> The unique function of the nurse is to assist the individual (sick or well), in the performance of those activities contributing to health or its recovery (or to peaceful death) that he would perform unaided if he had the necessary strength, will, or knowledge. And to do this in such a way as to help him gain independence as rapidly as possible.

Henderson also emphasized the need to determine the best approaches for answering questions about nursing practice. There was a need to define nursing and to incorporate its essential content in a meaningful way into programs of nursing education. This need placed an inherent responsibility on the nurse faculty member to develop increased knowledge about clinical phenomena.

The strongly felt need to bring nursing practice and education closer, as well as to develop a system (or model) for nursing practice (Smith, 1964), was addressed by Dorothy Smith at the University of Florida in the 1950s when she assumed the dual positions of director of nursing in the service setting and dean in the educational setting. This approach, which she took in 1959, was, perhaps, needed as a first step in the process of dealing with the fragmentation, which had developed in nursing as a whole. Since the initiation of this joint appointment, a number of different approaches have been introduced to deal with the division of service and education, with one of the most recent being the organization of nurse-managed health care centers (Nichols, 1985).

Assumptions about Faculty Practice

The nurse faculty member is accountable for maintaining clinical skills, for nursing is an an applied discipline. These clinical skills, of course, will be focused on the individual's particular area of clinical interest and expertise. The faculty member is also accountable for teaching students along with the myriad responsibilities, which accompany the faculty role, i.e., community service, college or university service, professional service, scholarship, etc. Is the performance of this total role a realistic expectation? The answers to this question need to be carefully weighed in relation to each individual situation. Algase (1986) believes that, in order to make it possible for faculty to maintain clinical skills, their practice should be funded differently from their teaching functions. Appropriate funding for practice calls for some innovative ideas and approaches.

Before nursing proceeds further in emphasizing the faculty member's practice responsibilities along with the other responsibilities, there are some assumptions, which might be made about faculty practice. These assumptions should receive careful consideration from both nursing education and nursing service agencies as roles and funding for these roles are considered. Likewise, the individual nurse considering a collaborative appointment should use these assumptions as a guide for considering choices:

1. Faculty practice should not exist in isolation from students.
2. Faculty practice should include creative approaches based on an expert base of knowledge and skills.
3. Faculty practice should exist in a balanced relationship with other aspects of the faculty role.
4. Faculty practice should be funded from patient or client revenue, not from student revenue.

Faculty as Role Models

A major impetus for collaboration was that students have positive role models. Students can and do learn by observation. Expert role modeling provides students with examples, which they will probably want to imitate. Christman (1979a, p. 8) summarizes the need for role modeling as follows:

The role internalization that takes place during the education process greatly influences the final set of values and clinical behaviors that each nurse will portray during a lifetime of professional endeavors. Nursing students do not have the rich advantage for learning clinical style that students in the other major clinical professions enjoy. Students in other professions learn the parameters of the clinical model of care from the better practitioners in each profession. Nursing students, however, are placed in the invidious position of being caught frequently in the covert guerilla warfare between nursing staff and nursing faculty where the students are viewed as invaders and disrupters of care or, at best, tolerated with social politeness. Students, by default of the faculty, must use staff nurses as models of clinical practice. . . . The alienation of students from the profession may be one of the outcomes of this lack of expert behavioral modeling in nursing education.

Much has been written in recent years about nursing's image and nurses' image of themselves. The positive role modeling generated by the collaborative movement should assist in improving nursing's self-concept. As students are increasingly exposed to nurses who are fully functioning in the professional role, their own development should assume a truly professional orientation. When nurses view themselves in a positive manner, it is likely that the public will also.

Collaborative or unification models will emphasize role modeling as an approach to learning. It is an approach, which needs further exploration with an evaluation of outcomes, for it has received only limited attention in the past. In fact, nursing seems to have been more focused in the past on "eating its young," a focus formed by the attitude that "I learned by jumping into the fire, and so can you." The evaluation of a program's success should give much consideration to the question: Did students perceive faculty as role models in practice whom they desired to emulate? Even though role modeling is generally acknowledged as one of the major bonuses of faculty practice, little appears in the literature to document that this is actually the case.

Organizational Support for Role Modeling. There may be various approaches to achieving positive educational outcomes. A summary of some of the earlier organizational models is shown in Table 4–1, beginning with the University of Florida model of the late 1950s and progressing through the 1960s and early 1970s with the documented models at Case Western Reserve University, University of Rochester, and Rush University. Each of these four situations were somewhat different, but all focused on some degree of collaboration (Nayer, 1980). These models demonstrate that, if two agencies (service and education) desire collaboration, working out the mechanics does take a great deal of planning. In other words, there must be real commitment to the concept by all involved.

The University of Rochester unification model designates each faculty member as a Clinician II. Some may function in direct line positions in nursing service, while others may work in a staff relationship such as consultant. The Clinician IIs "serve as expert role models who are highly skilled and effective practitioners"

TABLE 4–1. EDUCATION–SERVICE COLLABORATION MODELS: SOME EXAMPLES

Sponsorship	Organizational Description
College of Nursing, University of Florida/University of Florida Hospital, Gainesville, Florida	Shared appointment provided leadership for both the educational and service settings. Dorothy Smith served as Dean, College of Nursing and Chief of Nursing Practice, University Hospital. Faculty served as role models through extended practice privileges.
School of Nursing, Case Western Reserve University/Case Western University Hospitals, Cleveland, Ohio	Collaboration between Dean, School of Nursing, and Administrator of Nursing Service. Same person serves as Chairperson of clinical area in both settings. Faculty hold nursing service appointments and some nursing service personnel hold faculty appointments. Additional joint appointments exist without cost sharing but with practice and research privileges.
School of Nursing, University of Rochester/University of Rochester Medical Center, Rochester, New York	Positions of Dean of the School of Nursing and Director of Nursing Service are held by the same person. Clinical chiefs in each clinical area are responsible for both practice and education in their areas; they work closely with associate deans who provide guidance. The staff nurse is a Clinician I. The faculty-clinician appointment is labeled as Clinician II. Collaboration is the overall method of functioning.
College of Nursing, Rush University/Rush-Presbyterian-St. Luke's Medical Center, Chicago, Illinois	Matrix organization: Decision-making is decentralized with accountability at each level. Offices of Dean, College of Nursing, and Director of Nursing Services are combined. Program directors have responsibility for specific programs. Chairpersons have responsibility for managing their assigned departments. Unit leaders are responsible for managing specific units. Teacher practitioners are self-directed professionals who interact with those in the matrix organization.

(Sovie, 1981a, p. 49). Each faculty member at Rush University plans and negotiates her own clinical experiences; clinical teaching with students is then matched with these. The planning and distribution of each faculty member's workload is deemed to be critical to the success of the teacher-practitioner role. It is felt that ''Nursing students must see the nursing role portrayed in its full panoply in order to appreciate the professional excitement it can generate'' (Christman, 1979a, p. 9).

Nurse-managed Centers. One of the most recent faculty practice arrangements is the nurse-managed center. A variety of centers have been reported in the literature; each has been developed to meet health care needs, as well as identified educational goals (Arlton & Miercort, 1980; Culbert-Hinthorn, Fiscella, & Shortridge, 1985; Duffy & Halloran, 1986; Ossler et al., 1982; Nichols, 1985; Ryan & Barger-Lux,

1985; Smith, 1986). See Table 4–2 for a summary of these. A nurse-managed center is defined as "a health care facility managed by nurses" (Nichols, p. 85). Again, these centers may take a variety of forms; the common element is the control of nursing practice by nurses. The obvious advantages are that an exemplary learning climate can be experienced by students and that nurses can create and study a

TABLE 4–2. NURSE-MANAGED CENTERS: SOME EXAMPLES

Sponsorship	Services	Clients
Catholic University of America School of Nursing Washington, D.C.	Community–community mental health: home visits for individual and family assessment, health instruction, and supervision of acute and chronic health problems	700 low-income residents in a residential complex
Creighton University School of Nursing Omaha, Nebraska	Home health care Preventive care Sickness care	Clients obtained through contracts with several public and social service agencies; includes a variety of age groups and health problems
	Health enrichment Preventive and wellness services Client teaching	175 elderly people in a residential facility
Metropolitan State College College of Nursing Denver, Colorado	Nursing clinic Health maintenance and illness prevention Management of acute and chronic illness	Voluntary participants in a senior citizens center
Pace University Lienhard School of Nursing New York, New York	Primary health care services Assessment Teaching Counseling Referral	Students enrolled on the Pleasantville (N.Y.) campus
University of Florida: College of Nursing Housing Division Student Health Services Gainesville, Florida	Primary health care services Assessment Teaching Counseling Referral	Student's spouses and children who are living in student housing
University of Wisconsin–Milwaukee School of Nursing Milwaukee, Wisconsin	Health promotion clinic for individuals and families undergoing stressful life changes	Families who have children with asthma and are having trouble making needed adjustments
Yale University School of Nursing New Haven, Connecticut	Full maternity care All prenatal care Labor and delivery coverage	Any maternity patient who seeks care

system in which professional nursing can be practiced. Such centers offer an alternative to learning environments, which have developed around the medical model, and which may allow little flexibility and creativity for innovative nursing practice. Some of the concerns related with the earlier collaborative appointments (identified above) do not exist within this type of practice arrangement.

Planning for a nurse-managed center begins with the identification of a needed health care service and the evaluation of this need to determine whether it is being met by existing agencies and whether it can be appropriately addressed by nurses. Goals are then set, focusing on the integration of service, education, and management. If the center is to provide a teaching-learning environment as well as nursing service, the type of student experiences to be provided must be determined. For example, the Clinical Practice Unit (CPU) at Pace University grew out of an initial need to provide student experiences in primary care when only limited clinical sites were available (Culbert-Hinthorn et al., 1985). The Nursing Clinic established at the Catholic University of America provided a clinical setting for undergraduate students for an integrated practicum in community–community health nursing (Ossler et al., 1982). The Yale Nurse–Midwifery Practice, while providing "guaranteed midwifery care at all points" during the reproductive cycle, also provided graduate students with the opportunity of experiencing a private practice environment and, within this, independent decision making (Nichols, 1985, p. 85).

Management goals in these nurse-managed centers focus on both (1) management of client's care and (2) operation of the center itself. Both foci can provide valuable student learning. Although this second focus has not been discussed generally in the literature, such centers could provide an excellent learning opportunity for students interested in management supportive of health care services. An initial management function involves decisions related to the administrative and financial support of the center. Pursuit of these tasks follows the identification of the service and educational goals. Support for some of the existing centers comes from a variety of sources. Development of this support, it seems, calls for creativity in looking into nontraditional approaches to funding and support. The Yale Nurse–Midwifery Practice is working towards becoming self-supporting, and it rents a clinic space in a hospital setting. "Low-key ads" are being used to increase the well-woman gynecology caseload, since this area is viewed as one which would make the practice more cost-effective (Nichols, 1985). The CPU at Pace University received funds from the Robert Wood Johnson Foundation for some initial start-up costs. The University provided space, utilities, maintenance, and insurance for the health facility itself (Culbert-Hinthorn et al., 1985). Certainly, the nurse-managed centers can provide an excellent learning experience in offering health care cost-effectively, for the hidden nursing costs, which exist in traditional health care agencies, do not exist here.

One of the current factors most strongly hampering development of such centers is the health care delivery system itself, which does not provide third-party reimbursement for nurses. This means that, generally, referral of clients will still need to come from physicians. When schools exist in medical centers, they can focus on the advantage of having residents and interns available for consultation and referral. This should also foster the development of a collaborative process in the provision of health care by nurses and physicians.

Overall, the nurse-managed centers avoid some of the disadvantages associated with the earlier collaborative models. Working out the organizational model still takes much creative planning. The challenge, though, of creating a new model rather than trying to fit nursing into a traditional medical-focused organization may be a more exciting one. Certainly, there is a greater degree of freedom and autonomy for studying nursing practice and reporting the findings. This approach may not be the panacea for assisting the faculty member to balance all of the different aspects of the professional role, but some of the known problems of working with the more traditional models can be addressed during the planning phase. The opportunities exist for the teacher practitioner to move forward in the development of innovative approaches. The basic requirement is a strong commitment to the identified goals by all involved.

Quality of Nursing Care

Another of the major advantages of the collaborative arrangement which is frequently mentioned is that the quality of nursing care increases. Quality, in any setting, is evaluated by how well standards are met. In the case of the educational institution, external standards are provided by the National League for Nursing (NLN) and regional accrediting agencies. In the clinical setting, external standards necessary for mandatory or voluntary accreditation are provided by such agencies as the Joint Commission for the Accreditation of Hospitals (JCAH), National League for Nursing, and state health departments. Optional standards for nursing services, such as those provided by the American Nurses' Association, are also available and provide excellent guidelines. Each individual professional nurse, regardless of primary orientation, is accountable for meeting agency standards. The teacher in the clinical setting also has a responsibility for assisting students to meet the standards of that agency.

A basic knowledge of the standards guiding both the educational and the service agencies is a must for the nurse who is working in both settings. This is basic to making the collaborative arrangement work. The faculty member incorporates this information into nursing content throughout the curriculum and uses it at appropriate times. An understanding of the clinical agency standards and how they are being put into practice is also helpful for students and faculty in interpreting why they may or may not participate in certain kinds of activities and to what degree they may participate. Likewise, an understanding of the educational agency's standards helps the nurse clinician understand why certain kinds of learning experiences are essential for students.

A look at some common examples, which occur as part of the teaching–learning experience, might be helpful. Each of these situations involves a case where procedures or protocols have been designed to meet designated nursing care standards. Evaluate, while reading each of the examples, how information about standards would have improved the situation. Think, also, about how each situation might have been improved if the faculty member had held a clinical agency appointment.

Situation 1

> The student is admitting a patient to the hospital for surgery the following day. She incorrectly signs as the witness on the operative consent form. This is discovered just as the patient (already sedated) goes to the operating room the next morning.

Situation 2

> The student is assigned to care for a patient who has had an IV in place for 48 hours. The unit manager becomes upset at time of change of shift when she realizes that the student has not changed the IV site.

Situation 3

> The faculty member and the student take a verbal order from a physician, write the order on the chart, and the faculty member signs it. The staff nurse questions the medication order and refuses to administer it.

Quite simply, these situations (which probably are not too atypical) would have had less chance of occurring if the faculty member understood the agency's standards and related policies and procedures. In situation 1, for example, the faculty member would certainly have known that a student could not legally sign a preoperative consent form if she held a current appointment in the clinical agency. Situation 2 could, likewise, have been avoided. The hospital's policy of changing the IV site at least every 48 hours is basic to its standard of "safe" nursing care. Situation 3 is a murky one. It would have been appropriate for the faculty member to take and sign the order only if he or she holds an appointment in the clinical agency. The staff nurse who questions the order's accuracy certainly should be hesitant about administering the medication. Whether the order is correct or not, quality is affected because the mistrust between the faculty and staff nurse is deepened and future cooperation is threatened. Communication, a key factor in quality control, should be enhanced by collaborative arrangements.

Promoting Quality through Collaboration. Committee participation is an excellent method of sharing faculty and clinicians. Having an educator serve on such clinical agency committees as the quality assurance committee, records committee, and procedures committee would be most helpful in relaying some of the information and avoiding some of the kinds of situations presented above. The input provided from another perspective, too, could be most valuable in improving nursing care. Likewise, having clinical agency representatives on the school's curriculum committee and other appropriate committees could be helpful in planning the best possible clinical learning experiences.

Quality assurance studies play an enormous role in the achievement of quality nursing care, and this should be a high-priority area for collaboration. While quality assurance studies represent one type of research, they are often categorized separately because they are such an essential part of meeting the agency's goals. Today, any studies of cost also need to look at quality. This, in fact, may be one of the most pressing areas of need for collaborative arrangements at the present time.

Summary

The concept of collaboration certainly has many advantages in the area of practice. It is basic to the advancement of nursing. Regardless of whether the primary orientation is service or education, nurses' working together as colleagues in the clinical area, giving guidance to future nurses, is the desirable approach for the ultimate improvement of nursing services. Working in a collaborative arrangement, however, does have risks. An awareness that these risks exist might assist the individual nurse to minimize them as he or she sets personal goals and adjusts priorities as demanded by the situation.

EDUCATION

Administrative Support

There must be strong administrative support from both the nursing education and nursing service agencies in order to make collaborative appointments workable. By no means should it be assumed that the arrangement of these appointments has been perfected. The following questions represent some of the concerns of those who have been involved in collaborative appointments:

1. To whom is the teacher practitioner responsible?
2. How is the salary negotiated and paid?
3. How is time spent between the two agencies negotiated?
4. Does patient care or education take priority when staffing is inadequate?
5. How can the time commitment for clinical practice be justified?
6. How is practice balanced with teaching and scholarly activities in decisions of tenure and promotion?
7. Does the time spent in clinical practice affect scholarly productivity?

These concerns cannot be taken lightly. Collaboration offers many positive benefits for nursing and the individual nurse; thus, it is deserving of nursing's best thought. To avoid burnout in collaborative roles, it is important that these questions be addressed and workable solutions identified. While the questions may be the same in most situations, the answers or solutions will depend upon the different variables involved.

The first question of responsibility is an important one. In most situations, these probably exist both formally and informally. For example, one teacher practitioner states:

> It was important for both the head nurse on my unit and the director of the undergraduate program to understand my practice and education commitments. But of the two, I felt my relationship with my head nurse/unit leader was more critical. In order to begin to think of educational responsibilities, I had to create a conducive climate for students on my unit. It was essential for the nursing staff to realize that the head nurse/unit leader and I were in agreement about my role on the unit and that we were supportive of each other's responsibilities (Holm, 1981, pp. 655–656).

The informal dilemma expressed here can become a problem in view of the fact that the teacher practitioner is not equally visible in both environments. If the undergraduate director of the school was the person ultimately evaluating the performance of this faculty member, this inherently could become a problem. The time and energy invested by this faculty member in creating a good relationship and learning environment within the clinical facility could possibly go unrecognized when she is evaluated for salary increase, tenure, and promotion.

This may lead to the question of whether there should be two types of appointments, e.g., tenure-track and non-tenure-track. Or does this question recycle back to the service-education division, which originally led to the need for collaborative appoinments?

Rutgers College of Nursing has responded to the potential problems related to tenure and promotion decisions with an individualized approach (Joel, 1985). They have achieved "manpower sharing" through three types of collaborative arrangements: clinical, associate, and shared appointments. None of these appointments involves any exchange of money. The clinical and associate appointments are made to nurses who work in the clinical agencies where Rutgers students have learning assignments and to faculty members, respectively. The shared arrangement is referred to as a "manpower exchange" because there is no money exchange. Faculty holding the shared appointment are selected primarily from tenured faculty members or, in some cases, those holding terminal degrees. This approach lessens some of the pressure for nontenured faculty members who are attempting to achieve the requirements for tenure.

When there is exchange of salary, it should be negotiated between the individual nurse and the two agencies involved. In order for a collaborative program to be successful in the university, it must be viewed positively by all involved. The conclusion of a study by one university faculty group states:

> However the issue of compensation for faculty practice is resolved, any plan must both provide faculty with the incentive to provide services and offer consumers the opportunity to have access to their expertise. This means that an economic system must be developed that allows for regular public scrutiny of its effectiveness and is responsive to that scrutiny, in that it can be modified as needed. Only under these

conditions can a meaningful faculty reimbursement plan be established (Smith, 1980, p. 676).

Such a plan should provide appropriate incentives and rewards for faculty practice. The mechanics of working out such a plan in a traditional health care setting, however, would offer a challenge. Plans for working out reimbursement models should be a high priority for any educational agency that commits itself to faculty practice. The client outcomes, as well as the faculty and student outcomes, should be evident.

Learning Climate

A truly collaborative model should narrow the education–service gap by creating an environment, which uses the best talents of all involved in a constructive manner. The creation of a better learning climate for students is a frequently acknowledged advantage of collaboration. This is difficult to objectively evaluate, but there are questions, which can be asked to determine whether the learning climate is a positive one. Affirmative answers to the following questions would indicate that this is occurring.

1. Are faculty and clinicians accepting each other as professional colleagues?
2. Does the practitioner teacher feel that he or she is experiencing a full professional role?
3. Is the practitioner teacher able to involve students, directly or indirectly, in practice?
4. Are nurses (regardless of whether primary orientation is clinical or teaching) involved in discovering or applying new knowledge?
5. Are all nurses involved in the evaluation of nursing services?
6. Is there an identifiable model of professional nursing practice?

The creation of a professional nursing practice model should be one of the real benefits gained through collaboration. It further enhances the learning environment for students. If there is such a model in place, this should be identifiable to the student through a variety of observations such as the following:

1. The standards of nursing care are reflected in all phases of care: assessment, diagnosis, planning, intervention, and evaluation.
2. Clients are involved in identifying their own health care needs and problems and setting individual goals.
3. Excellent client and family teaching programs and materials are being used.
4. Nursing research activity is evident through ongoing studies, as well as the utilization of findings in practice.
5. Nurses are involved in working with other health care professionals (through research, committee participation, etc.) in designing new and innovative approaches to health care.

Summary

If the educational arena truly believes that it is essential for the faculty member to be involved in practice, then educational institutions must be willing to continue to explore workable collaborative arrangements. This will require that additional models be tried and evaluated. Some of the major areas that need to be addressed as schools and clinical agencies continue to work towards collaboration include:

1. Identification of appropriate incentives and rewards, including how the payment of salary should be administratively handled.
2. Weight, which practice should carry in relation to teaching, service, and scholarly activities, in decisions of merit, promotion, and tenure.
3. Organizational arrangement, which clearly identifies the person(s) to whom the practitioner teacher is responsible.
4. Evaluation procedures, which address the variety of contributions made by the practitioner teacher.

RESEARCH

Collaborative efforts provide a mechanism for increasing nurses' involvement in practice-oriented research at a time when health care is changing so rapidly. Research efforts are needed in a variety of areas, including clinical nursing practice, cost-effective approaches to practice, patient-client outcomes, and testing nursing theories. The joint ventures between service and education will, hopefully, have the effect of creating a "spirit of inquiry" within nursing students and all nurses, regardless of primary work orientation. This research involvement is the very fiber of nursing; it provides the framework for moving the profession forward. "Generating a scientific basis for nursing practice is crucial to provision of quality care to clients as well as to the design and assessment of innovative models for health care delivery" (Brimmer et al., 1983, p. 165).

The decade of the 1980s promises to show a great deal of progress in the development of nursing knowledge. Collaboration between the nurse researcher and the nurse clinician, with the associated role modeling for students, is offering a positive approach to both the generation and utilization of the knowledge needed for practice.

Administrative Support for Research

The nurse administrator's belief in the importance of research for clinical and administrative decision making is essential to the successful initiation of a research program in the clinical setting. This importance is explained by Chance and Hinshaw (1980, p. 32):

> Establishing a research program requires a commitment of resources and time. Basic to such a commitment is a belief that sound administrative and clinical

decisions for nursing practice must be based on accurate data. However, administrative and clinical staff must be aware of the risks involved with research, the data may not show desired results or may not be clearly interpretable.

If the administrator values research and is accepting of the fact that results may not always support a desired position, then the nursing staff will be more likely to value and become involved in research.

Certainly, the support for research must come from all nurses in the clinical agency if a successful program is to be created. One of the first investments of resources may be directed towards staff development for research participation. This is an area where collaborative arrangements can be most helpful, using the talents of those with expertise in research methodology. Often, such a person's primary involvement is in the educational setting. Educational activities (formal and informal) can be provided to assist nurses in becoming involved in research activities, as well as in valuing the effects of research on their practice.

During the past several years, there has been a move to place nursing research within the clinical agency's formal organizational framework (Chance & Hinshaw, 1980; Cronenwett, 1986; Hoare & Earenfight, 1986). The placement of research in the agency's formal organization might take any one of the following approaches, which have been described in the literature: (1) a department of nursing research with a nurse serving as associate director for nursing research, (2) research responsibilities included in the clinical nurse specialist's job description, (3) a unit-based approach using designated research facilitators, and (4) a department of nursing development and research with a nurse coordinator acting as liaison between this department and the department of nursing. The first three approaches seem preferable, since they place the direct responsibility for nursing research within the department of nursing. The last is least desirable, for coordination between nursing and other departments can be achieved through informal activities rather than through a formal organizational structure, which places the position outside of nursing.

Any one of these approaches, though, presents a viable option for the faculty member who desires to collaborate with the clinical agency with a focus on research activities. In addition to considering their respective goals, the nurse and the agency might look at some of the functions, which have been identified in the literature as appropriate for such a position:

1. Guiding the design of practice-oriented research studies.
2. Providing staff development through formal classes and workshops.
3. Providing staff development through informal individual and group guidance at the unit level.
4. Assisting nurses to state problems identified in nursing practice as researchable problem statements.
5. Consulting with nurses related to the variety of investigative roles they might assume.
6. Identifying and developing strategies to increase and intensify research activities within the agency.

7. Participating in the establishment of guidelines for the protection of human subjects in research.
8. Serving on the agency's research committee.
9. Considering ways of sharing significant research findings.
10. Coordinating efforts for the sharing of research findings.
11. Seeking available resources and funding for research.
12. Interacting with nurse faculty members in the clinical agency in relation to shared research goals.
13. Facilitating the research studies, which are performed by students within the agency setting.
14. Collecting and organizing research-related resources (books, journals, reports, etc.) for nursing staff members.
15. Promoting utilization of existing research findings as appropriate.

A variety of resources are needed to carry out these research functions. Cronenwett (1986) has identified those resources listed below as essential, and these provide a basis for determining the agency's commitment to supporting an active research program.

1. Time
2. Space
3. Secretarial support
4. Library facilities
5. Equipment and supplies
6. Monetary support for computer time, coding and data entry, reproduction of instruments, travel for paper presentation
7. Access to expert consultants
8. Access (which might involve travel) to professional peers

A collaborative arrangement provides the advantage of cost sharing. For example, most clinical agencies do not have the type of computer services available to provide for the statistical analysis of data. This is available, though, through the university computer services. Universities also provide needed library resources. In some instances, both agencies may share in support of travel.

Research as a Teaching Strategy

If research is seen as a way of increasing the professionalization of nursing, then nursing education must find a way of socializing students into the role of researcher or user of nursing knowledge. Whether or not time is allotted to learning about research carries an important message to students, just as the nurse administrator's willingness to provide time for research activity carries an important message to the practicing nurse.

Faculty do have a responsibility for involving both undergraduate and graduate students in research. A number of different teaching strategies can be used with both: (1) critiquing research study reports, (2) relating research findings to clinical nursing topics discussed, (3) discussing research results, which relate to the planning of care for an individual client, and (4) questioning some of nursing's undying "rituals" (which students might be motivated to try to lay to rest). While these students may not have a real understanding of statistics at the undergraduate level, they can begin to value the applications of research to practice.

Research itself can be used as a teaching strategy. Although this is just one reason why it is important for faculty and clinicians to be personally involved in research, it emphasizes the real relevance of research for practice. Students can be involved in the actual research process in a number of ways: (1) discussing the planning, implementation, and evaluation of the study with the researchers; (2) collection of data; (3) analysis of data; and (4) analyzing the effectiveness of the research design. This approach is probably most applicable for teaching graduate students. Again, role modeling is an effective method of teaching. Role modeling as a technique for teaching research methods to nursing faculty was shown to be more effective than small group discussion (Kramer, Holaday, & Hoeffer, 1981).

Practice-oriented Research

A practice-oriented research program in nursing is directed towards four major areas: clinical nursing, administration, evaluation, and utilization (Chance & Hinshaw, 1980). Clinical nursing studies have direct concern with and applicability for practice. Research questions arise from practice and might address nursing interventions or client outcomes. Nursing administration studies might focus on a variety of problems related to the management of patient care, i.e., cost of nursing care, staff turnover, nurse satisfaction, and staffing patterns. Needed decisions concerning the delivery of nursing care direct the questions to be investigated. Evaluative studies address the effectiveness of such ongoing programs within nursing as quality control and staff development. These studies are guided primarily by the need to document the quality of nursing care provided. The utilization portion of the program focuses on the use of research results by nursing staff members. It involves both facilitating staff's use of research findings as well as evaluating the outcomes of this use of prior research.

The Conduct and Utilization of Research in Nursing (CURN) was a 5-year research development project in Michigan, which developed a Collaborative Research Program (CRP) model for carrying out practice-oriented research. This model "included direct involvement of clinicians as team members during every phase of the research process." It was felt that, by involving clinicians in the formulation of the study's research questions and design, "more practice-relevant clinical nursing research would result" (Krone & Loomis, 1982, p. 38). The CURN project has increased interest in collaborative arrangements between researchers and clinicians. The recommendations for nursing administrators interested in working out such arrangements, based on the implementation of this project, were "Allow clinicians adequate time to devote to the project" and "Provide a 'resource link' to help clinicians find research partners" (pp. 40–41). The CRP did demonstrate the success of combining the efforts and expertise of nurse researchers and clinicians. It is an approach for closing the gap between service and research.

The CURN recommendations provide a "reasonable model for bonding education and practice through research" (Lancaster, 1984, p. 379). Research can assist in closing the gap between service and education. Educators need access to clinical settings in order to carry out practice-oriented research. They may also need the validation of their research questions or "hunches" by nurses practicing in the setting. While clinicians have questions related to their practice, they may lack the skills in research methodology needed to carry out a study. Working together to carry out a research study, to which each can bring her interest and expertise, is an excellent example of how nurses in service and education settings can work together to improve nursing practice.

Summary

Research provides promise as a vehicle for integrating practice and education. In addition, research will move the profession forward through the validation and generation of nursing knowledge. It provides the common ground on which nursing will continue to build.

Research provides a logical place for practice and education to collaborate. The practice-oriented studies, which are a high priority in nursing, call for the combined expertise of educators, clinicians, and researchers (whatever their primary work orientation might be). The resources needed to carry out research can best be provided jointly by service and educational agencies. The research questions generate from practice, and the clinical agency provides access to the sample population. More generally, the university is better able to supply such resources as library and computer access, programs, and consultation.

In order to make a collaborative arrangement workable, there has to be a high degree of commitment from the nursing administrators in both the educational and service setting, as well as from the individual nurse involved. Such arrangements will be enhanced as research becomes more valued by all nurses in both settings.

CONSULTATION

In combination with practice, education, and research, consultation rounds out the full professional role. It lends itself very naturally to collaboration, for consultative arrangements usually evolve between service and education agenices when specific areas of need are identified. Consultative assistance may be requested from an identified person or group who has the expertise to share. Agencies might even formalize a system for facilitating consultation; for example, a helpful approach is the publication of a list of nurses, by each agency, noting the specific areas in which each would be willing to provide consultation.

Consultation probably fits most often within the associate type of appointment; that is, there may be sharing of expertise between agencies with no exchange of money. This may be referred to as a "reciprocal" relationship. For faculty members, sharing their expertise with service agencies may fall into the "service" area.

This means that when they are evaluated on the major areas of "teaching," "scholarship," and "service," the donation of their time and expertise to the clinical agency is noted within the latter area.

One faculty group (University of Connecticut) devleoped a unique type of collaborative arrangement, which they called a "clinical consultancy" (Polifroni & Schmalenberg, 1985). This was a "consulting" relationship, which was established to meet the goal of keeping faculty involved in the practice setting, and, which was located 40 miles from campus. "Consultancy" was interpreted, in this case, to include faculty functioning in the following roles: "direct patient care, role modeling, inservice education, projects, information resource, and head nurse support" (p. 227). The program allowed faculty to spend one day a week in the clinical setting (without student responsibilities); reimbursement was provided by that agency.

In addition to the methods (committee participation, providing staff education, collaborating with clinicians on research projects, etc.), which have been previously mentioned within the practice, education, and research aspects of the professional role, a consulting arrangement may be negotiated between the individual or group and the agency who wishes to employ these services. This may occur at any specified time, rather than on the continuing basis, which occurs with the associate or shared appointment. Most universities allow faculty to carry out some consulting in addition to performance of the faculty role, if this does not interfere with overall performance. Some schools may set a limitation on the amount of time, which can be spent in such activities. Nurse faculty who enter into this type of negotiation must be willing to put a "price" on their knowledge and skills. Nurses, in the past, have been very hesitant to do this. As the nurse experiences the full development of the professional role, however, this should become, not only more acceptable, but also more comfortable.

CONCLUSION

Faculty practice and research is not only desirable; in many situations, it is now an expectation. Nurse faculty need to experience the full professional role, which is interpreted to include practice, education, research, and consultation. If a faculty member is functioning in a collaborative arrangement, then he or she is probably performing, to some degree, within all four of these areas. Priorities of the individual may continue to change as professional goals are continuously evaluated and refined. It is important to recognize that, realistically, one person cannot perform all of these roles equally at a given time.

Numerous advantages and disadvantages of collaboration have been discussed. There is no one perfect arrangement, which will fit all situations, though there are now a number of tested models available to serve as guides. Each situation must consider the goals of the agencies and the individual nurse involved. Then serious negotiation should include consideration of some of the known pitfalls of joint appointments. The positive outcomes still outweigh the problems of working out such an arrangement. Flexibility and a willingness to change must be a key ingredient of all involved.

There continues to be a gap between nursing service and education; collaborative nursing roles do provide one mechanism for narrowing it. As the profession works towards this goal, however, nurses must realize that some diversity needs to be maintained. The goal should never be to put all nurses into the same mold; rather, it should be to assist nurses to develop different strengths and then to blend these strengths for the best of the whole of nursing. The profession can use the interests, strengths, and best efforts of all.

REFERENCES

Algase, D. L. (1986). Faculty practice: A means to advance the discipline of nursing. *Journal of Nursing Education, 25*(2), 74–76.

Arlton, D. M., & Miercort, O. S. (1980). A nursing clinic: The challenge for student learning opportunities. *Journal of Nursing Education, 19*(1), 53–58.

Brimmer, P. F., Skoner, M. M., Pender, N. J., Williams, C. A., Fleming, J. W., & Werley, H. H. (1983). Nurses with doctoral degrees: Education and employment characteristics. *Research in Nursing and Health, 6*(4), 157–165.

Chance, H. C., & Hinshaw, A. S. (1980). Strategies for initiating a research program. *Journal of Nursing Administration, 10*(3), 32–39.

Christman, L. (1979a). The practitioner-teacher. *Nurse Educator, 4*(2), 8–11.

Christman, L. (1979b). On the scene: Uniting service and education at Rush-Presbyterian-St. Luke's Medical Center. *Nursing Administration Quarterly, 3*(3), 7–40.

Cronenwett, L. R. (1986). Research reflections: The research role of the clinical nurse specialist. *Journal of Nursing Administration, 16*(4), 10–11.

Culbert-Hinthorn, P., Fiscella, K. D., & Shortridge, L. M. (1985). A nurse-managed clinical practice unit: Part I—the positives. *Nursing and Health Care, 6*(2), 96–100.

Duffy, D. M., & Halloran, M. C. (1986). Meeting the challenge of multiple academic roles through a nursing center practice model. *Journal of Nursing Education, 25*(2), 55–58.

Henderson, V. (1966). *The nature of nursing.* New York: Macmillan.

Hicks, B. C., & Westphal, M. (1977). Integration of clinical and academic nursing at the hospital clinical unit level. *Journal of Nursing Education, 16*(4), 6–9.

Hinshaw, A. S., Chance, H. C., & Atwood, J. (1981). Research in practice: A process of collaboration and negotiation. *Journal of Nursing Administration, 11*(2), 33–38.

Hoare, K., & Earenfight, J. (1986). Unit-based research in a service setting. *Journal of Nursing Administration, 16*(4), 35–39.

Holm, K. (1981). Faculty practice—noble intentions gone awry? *Nursing Outlook, 29*(11), 655–657.

Joel, L. A. (1985). The Rutgers experience: One perspective on service–education collaboration. *Nursing Outlook, 33,* 220–224.

Kramer, K., Holaday, B., & Hoeffer, B. (1981). The teaching of nursing research—Part III: A comparison of teaching strategies. *Nurse Educator, 6*(2), 18–28.

Krone, K. P., & Loomis, M. E. (1982). Developing practice-relevant research: A model that worked. *Journal of Nursing Administration, 12*(4), 38–41.

Lancaster, J. (1984). Bonding of nursing practice and education through research. *Nursing and Health Care, 5*(8), 379–382.

Larson, E. (1981). Nursing research outside academia: A panel presentation. *Image, 13*(3), 75–77.
MacPhail, J. (1983). Collaboration/unification models for nursing education and nursing service. In Chaska, N. L. (Ed.), *The nursing profession: A time to speak* (pp. 637–649). New York: McGraw-Hill.
Nayer, D. D. (1980). Unification: Bringing nursing service and nursing education together. *American Journal of Nursing, 80*(6), 1110–1114.
Nichols, C. (1985). Faculty practice: Something for everyone. *Nursing Outlook, 33*(2), 85–90.
Nightingale, F. (1884). *Notes on nursing: What it is, and what it is not.* New York: D. Appleton and Company.
Ossler, C. C., Goodwin, M. E., Mariani, M., & Gilliss, C. L. (1982). Establishment of a nursing clinic for faculty and student clinical practice. *Nursing Outlook, 30*(7), 402–405.
Polifroni, E. C., & Schmalenberg, C. (1985). Faculty practice that works: Two examples. *Nursing Outlook, 33*(5), 226–228.
Powers, M. J. (1976). The unification model in nursing. *Nursing Outlook, 24*(4), 482–487.
Redman, B. K., Cassells, J. M., & Jackson, S. S. (1985). Generic baccalaureate nursing programs: Survey of enrollment, administrative structure/funding, faculty teaching/practice roles, and selected curriculum trends. *Journal of Professional Nursing, 1*(6), 369–380.
Ryan, S. A., & Barger-Lux, M. J. (1985). Faculty expertise in practice—a school succeeding. *Nursing and Health Care, 6*(2), 74–78.
Schlotfeldt, R. M., & MacPhail, J. (1969). An experiment in nursing: Implementing planned change. *American Journal of Nursing, 69*(7), 1475–1480.
Smith, D. M. (1964). Myth and method in nursing practice. *American Journal of Nursing, 64*(2), 68–72.
Smith, D. M. (1965). Education and service under one administration. *Nursing Outlook, 13*(2), 54–56.
Smith, E. M. (1986). A nurse-managed family health center at the University of Florida. *Journal of Nursing Education, 25*(2), 79–81.
Smith, G. R. (1980). Compensating faculty for their clinical practice. *Nursing Outlook, 28*(11), 673–676.
Sovie, M. D. (1981a). Unifying education and practice: One medical center's design. Part I. *Journal of Nursing Administration, 11*(1), 41–49.
Sovie, M. D. (1981b). Unifying education and practice: One medical center's design. Part II. *Journal of Nursing Administration, 11*(2), 30–32.
Staff (1985). "Consider this . . . collaboration pays off." *Journal of Nursing Administration, 15*(2), 4.

5

Productivity and Workloads

Margaret Denise Zanecchia, Ph.D., R.N.

One of the most important issues facing the nursing profession in the 1980s and 1990s is the mastery and implementation of the economic concepts necessary for its survival. Nursing education is not unique. Challenging tasks exist for nursing's educational leaders related to fiscal accountability. Questions are being raised by nursing educators regarding the realities of the program budget, productivity of faculty, and faculty workload measurement.

Because of declining federal support for higher education in nursing, increasing higher education costs, and a decreasing student applicant group, the economic survival of nursing education in the college system is becoming a critical situation. Some academic nursing programs have been closed, and some nursing faculty have lost jobs due to these reasons. However, a few new programs continue to open.

Understanding faculty productivity in the academic setting is important. Documentation for the quantitative and qualitative workload activities is one strategy for nursing educators. The pragmatic task is securing the data necessary for administrative decision making based on the meaning of a reasonable workload. Teaching load measured in numbers of students, classroom hours, and other faculty workload responsibilities increased significantly in the 1970s to 1980s, especially in the public sector (Minter & Bowen, 1982).

Often, nursing workloads have been higher than those in other academic disciplines. How much more load can be absorbed while faculty maintain the quality of their teaching? There are no indications that research and scholarly activities will become any less important than they have been in the past or are now.

One of the continuing problems, which has confronted nursing educators is the integrated collegiate program. Also, the team teaching model further complicates calculation of faculty workload. A part of the problem has been determining productivity for the workload of nurse educators involved in teaching in the clinical laboratory.

While other academic disciplines document faculty workloads in lecture and laboratory credit hours, nursing deans are tasked to refute the additional teaching hours necessary for clinical nursing laboratories. The 1 hour to 3 hour ratio has been used for computing the clinical credit hour. One lecture hour is equivalent to 3 clinical laboratory hours. Another possible ratio is 1 : 2. A specific ratio has not been required by the nursing accrediting organization, the National League for Nursing (NLN). However, the number of students with a faculty member in the clinical area can vary from 1 : 8 to 1 : 12, depending on the level of the student.

The Interacting System Model (ISM) suggests an organizing framework for the nurse educator in viewing the workload imposed by the multiple roles. The ISM uses the concepts of input and output to explain nursing faculty productivity. The nurse educator with educational degrees and teaching experience is considered as input. In addition, the other personnel resources in the nursing program, i.e., the secretarial and media personnel, are input.

A simple definition of productivity is the ratio of output to input. Workload is all activities that produce output (Templin, 1983, p. 2). Inputs are also the number of other faculty teaching the courses of the curriculum and performing all of the other roles.

Productivity Definitions
- *Workload:* All activities that produce output.
- *Productivity:* Ratio of input to output.
- *SCHG:* The number of students multiplied by number of credit hours taught in an academic year.
- *FTE:* The number of full-time faculty needed to teach the curriculum aside from other workload.
- *Ratio of productivity:* The number of credit hours generated per faculty to the total credit hours for all students divided by the total faculty.

ENVIRONMENT AND PRODUCTIVITY

Environmental factors that affect faculty productivity are related to:

- The forces in environment
- The faculty
- The division of work and responsibility
- The supervision of the work
- The administration

Both product and productivity also influence the environment. Products and productivity can be modified through the feedback loop of the open college system.

A productivity-centered work environment is one that has quality education as the goal. Regardless, limiting circumstances exist. An example is a shrinking 18-

year-old cohort. The need for an educational program with faculty and staff resources can be determined. However, vacillating budgets and other economic forces affect the number of faculty. The product outcomes (student learning) can also be affected.

Every college or university uses resources in the form of labor, capital, and nondurable supplies. Labor or personnel is primarily the faculty workload. The environment includes the facilities it provides, expectations it communicates, behavior it rewards, ways its members relate, and its policies, procedures, and programs (Pace, 1979).

Capital includes the buildings and equipment. The supplies and nondurable services include stationery, books, fuel, chemicals, etc. All of these resources are designed to produce learning through instruction, research, and public service. The interchange of inputs and resources produces educational output and probably societal changes (Bowen, 1977, p. 11).

Moos (1979) studied a variety of educational environments. Three types of environmental characteristics exist. The characteristics of an environment relate to:

- Its purpose
- Its human relationships
- Its management

The educational environment needs to be conducive to the institution's goals for student learning.

Productivity involves the effective management of resources, and processes to achieve specified objectives (Dressel, 1976, p. 85).

Faculty Workload and Productivity

Faculty productivity is viewed as a part of institutional productivity. Teaching productivity of faculty departments makes up the total institution's teaching workload. Faculty teaching productivity includes instructional processes and curriculum and course development.

Faculty productivity may be categorized as either individual or program output. Individual outputs for the nurse educator are teaching research, publications service, and increased self-worth. Faculty awards and professional recognition are given for increased productivity. The rewards for output are the successful students who meet course objectives, faculty promotions, tenure, and merit awards.

Faculty productivity may be assessed through:

- Teaching effectiveness
- Faculty research
- Faculty-created instructional materials
- Faculty advising
- Professional development
- Committee work

Program output includes the teaching of students through the curriculum process. Student outcomes, therefore, are increased knowledge and the deriving of a basis for social change. More difficult to measure, preparation for employment as a generalist or specialist is the student outcome of collegiate nursing programs.

Administrators of educational programs have more recently become concerned about the documentation of faculty productivity. Quantitative measures of teaching productivity (i.e., number of hours of instruction, number of students, and the number of credits earned) have been inadequate measures (Henderson & Henderson, 1974, p. 148). The question is both how much teaching and how to measure the teaching output. Defining faculty workload activities and measuring the outputs of education have been a challenge to higher education throughout the twentieth century.

Teaching, research, public service and some levels of administration have been a part of faculty activity since the 1920s. A distinction was made between teaching time and time spent in noninstructional activities (Koos, 1919).

In general, *faculty workload* by definition is the sum of all activities that take the time of a college or university teacher. The workload of faculty is related either directly or indirectly to professional responsibilities and interests of the faculty (Stickler, 1960, p. 80). Such a broad definition includes literally every activity of the nurse educator.

FACULTY WORKLOAD ACTIVITIES

There are many activities, which can definitely be included as faculty workload. Some activities are considered workload by some and not by others, i.e., general reading, participation in student discussions, and participation in faculty discussions. Individual research, consulting, public service functions, and advising student organizations are direct workload. Attending seminars, writing a textbook, and writing an article are types of indirect faculty workload, but may be included as faculty development and scholarly activity. The following is a listing of faculty workload activities:

- Actual teaching
- Preparation for teaching
- Writing examinations
- Correcting examinations
- Reading and grading papers
- Supervision in clinical and skills laboratories
- Consultation (nonpayment)
- Research or creative work
- Consulting (fee-generating)
- Directing graduate theses and dissertations
- Scholarship
- Professional services
- Interacting with students
- Advising students

- Counseling and guidance activities
- Administrative tasks
- Attending faculty meetings

Tenure is a predictor of faculty productivity (Murphy, 1978) and productivity is affected by certain attributes of the faculty, not only the years of teaching experience of the faculty, but also the teaching workload, research, and publications (Centra, 1980).

Three types of productivity measures were suggested for faculty: publications, use of a citation index, and the listings of faculty awards and honors. The citation index is an indicator of the impact of an article as measured by the number of times that colleagues had cited a particular faculty work (Holzemer, 1982).

Defining workload and productivity continues to challenge nursing educators. A model for faculty productivity focuses more on well-being, faculty role perception, and motivation. More faculty productivity exists when programs in faculty evaluation, faculty development, and collaborative administration are present (Andreoli & Musser, 1984).

Although multiple types of workload exist, nursing faculty workload is categorized as:

- Teaching workload
- Research workload
- Service workload
- Professional development workload
- Practice workload
- Advising workload

Teaching Workload

College teaching workload is defined in a variety of ways. Credit hour, student contact hour, student credit hours generated, or faculty clock hours may be utilized as a measure of faculty teaching workload.

Workweek Hours. The expected workweek of college faculty for many years was 35 clock hours. The average workload was 12 class hours, assuming 2 hours of preparation for each hour spent in class. Total workload is also calculated as the total number of hours, which the faculty work in a given week. The range is 45 to 57 hours per week. The minimum is probably 50 hours per week during the academic year. If the total number of hours were spread over a 48-week year with a 4-week vacation, it would amount to approximately 40 hours per week for a calendar year, assuming the 35-week academic year.

The amount of time spent per week at work varies greatly for the nursing academician. No two work weeks are exactly alike. The time varies with: the number of classes, amount of clinical preparation, number of student conferences and student evaluations, nursing department committee meetings, library reading, research, and participation in student and faculty activities.

Most nursing academics typically report working 40 to 60 hours in a week but this includes some research efforts or consulting. A difficult question often posed regards extra income-producing activities. Whether or not to consider these activities as part of the regular workload of the faculty is a problem. If faculty exceed an amount of discretionary time or if these activities detract from the workload hours available for research or public service, concern exists (Marsh, 1979). The current estimate for the average university nurse faculty is approximately 56 hours a week time on task. This includes the various roles of faculty and workload activities (Young, 1985, p. 332). Most universities have established guidelines for outside work not to exceed a certain percentage or 8 hours per week during the contract period.

Credit Hour. The workload of a nursing faculty member is often described in terms of the number of credit hours taught. Most programs use a 12-hour credit load, but some have loads of 9 credit hours, 6 credit hours, or even less. But this distinction is often made for those teaching in doctoral or graduate programs versus baccalaureate programs.

A constant ratio exists between credit-hour load and total load, so that credit-hour load gives a more reliable index of the total load (Stickler, 1960). If one asks how many credit hours the faculty teach per week, the answer usually ranges between 3 and 15, with the mode around 6 and 12 (Bogue, 1972).

Attempts are made to establish a more reliable measure of faculty workload called the scheduled credit hour, (SCH). The SCH/FTE was defined as the number of student credit hours taught by the faculty members' unit divided by the number of full-time-equivalent faculty in that unit. The advantages of a standardized workload measure are comparisons across departments, programs, schools, or universities. Other advantages are usefulness in budget planning and cost calculations. (Yuker, 1984, p. 10)

Teaching workload measured by scheduled credit hours generated (SCHG) was a variable in a study by Zanecchia (1981). An average mean for SCHG is approximately 100 SCHG per semester per faculty group. The mean SCHG was 183 hours for an academic year among 625 nursing faculty in 25 baccalaureate faculty groups in five programs over a 5-year period of time.

Contact Hour. Contact hours are used as a basis for defining loads. Yuker (1974) found contact hours to be a better criteria than credit hours. Contact hours defined as the 45 to 50 minute hour reflected work time rather than the arbitrary time indicated by credit hours (Yuker, 1984, p. 10).

Contact hours include adjustments for laboratory classes as courses that meet more or less than the stated number of credit hours. Currently, the contact hour seems to have become a more reliable measure of workload of faculty. The average range is 17 to 20 hours per week.

Percent Teaching Time. The percent of teaching time is yet another measure used to assess workload. No one, however, has been able to demonstrate whether collecting faculty load information by hours worked per unit of time is more accurate than percentage allocation of time. Needless to say, a warning must be given to those who would compare percentages when the base number of hours worked per week are different.

Undergraduate teaching, as the college mission, determines faculty workload across disciplines and in most types of institutions. Regardless of the professor's rank, age, sex, or the subject matter, undergraduate teaching is the work of the college faculty. Undergraduate teaching time averages 52 percent for general college faculty, while the average time spent in graduate education is 12 percent (Baldridge et al., 1978).

In nursing, teaching has comprised 70 to 75 percent of the faculty workload (Solomons, Jordison, & Powell, 1980). Defining faculty productivity in teaching is a difficult task. How the teaching is quantified and how productivity is measured is the subject of faculty–administration and administration–union debates. When the input–outcome model is utilized, quality, unfortunately, cannot be accurately measured.

The undergraduate teaching workload can be divided into seven methods of instruction: lecture, laboratory, discussion, seminar, independent study, tutorial, and programmed instruction. The associated activities of actual instruction include preparation time, from 2 to 3 hours outside the classroom for every hour of instruction and evaluation.

Teaching loads are sometimes reduced by agreement to allow for a variety of activities. These include such responsibilities as department chairperson, administrative responsibilities, a research grant, publishing as an author or co-author, the development of new courses or curriculum, services, developmental activities, special assignments, serving as acting chairperson of a standing committee, serving as officer in the faculty senate, serving as officer in a professional association, or engaging in legal activities for the profession (Goeres, 1978).

Productive Days. Teaching workload for faculty in general has also been described in terms of productive days per year per faculty member. Holliman (1977) analyzed nursing faculty workload for an academic year. The total nonproductive time was 143 days. This included days for vacation (20), for illness (5), for weekends (104), and for holidays (14). The remaining 225 productive days were designated as: 5, attendance at workshops; 9, committee work (at 6 hours per month); 20 for preparation of curriculum; 6 for advising students; 5 for faculty meetings; and 180 for class and clinical preparation.

A standard unit was suggested as an alternative measure of faculty teaching workload (Saylor et al., 1979). A standard of 40 units of work per week per semester was set. This standard could be met by teaching four undergraduate classes of 25 or fewer students for 3 class hours per week; or two undergraduate courses for 20 units, research for 10 units, and service for 10 units. The usual work week was

55.5 hours. Each program must, however, establish an individualized workload measuring system, which serves the faculty member, the department, and the institution.

Research Workload

Research workload has more recently become an integral part of the faculty workload. Only a few faculty were prepared for research in the early 1950s. For nursing, the research work as a faculty member is less well defined and poorly integrated into the total measurable faculty workload.

Nursing leaders encouraged research as a part of the professional role in the 1960s (Abdellah & Levine, 1965). By 1970, the American Nurses' Association had established a commission on nursing research, and in 1972, a Council of Nurse Researchers was formed (Young, 1985, p. 284). The emphasis on research as a part of the nursing faculty workload was established in the later 1970s.

Research and scholarly activity may be considered workload. All tasks, which are scholarly or are directed toward the scholarly pursuit of goals, are not defined as research, however.

The writing of books, articles, or reviews of writings relevant to professional nursing is scholarly productivity. Also, reviewing the work of a colleague or conducting inquiry and research is scholarly. Shils (1972) judged an activity as creative research and scholarship if it would lead to a solution that received an evaluation and critique by qualified peers. Publication in a scholarly journal guarantees a peer review. It is also a way to share findings with professional colleagues.

Other activities, which have been considered scholarship, are publications as editor or contributing author. Books or chapters that report research are ranked higher than nonresearch-related books. Articles in both refereed journals and non-refereed journals published on research or nonresearch are scholarly endeavors. Publishing in the newspapers of professional organizations further describes the faculty's scholarly activity.

Funded research grants are scholarly work. Research conducted without benefit of grant support is also scholarly. Whether the research study or grant is done on an individual basis or as part of a group effort, it is scholarly production. However, group research should not exist to the exclusion of individual research.

Sharing research findings at scholarly meetings held locally, regionally, or nationally is determined scholarly. The faculty who supervises students or directs peers in the research protocol is certainly demonstrating scholarly capacity. Participation in research colloquia or seminars is another type of research presentation. However, faculty attendance at research presentations, although scholarly, is on a lower level than the previously described activities.

Creative endeavors are considered to be scholarly activities, i.e., project, instructional media, course designs, program development, new curricula, or teaching modalities. Scholarly awards and recognition received by faculty are included in this workload category.

Research Time. The amount of faculty time devoted to research activity has varied throughout the years with the type of institution. Research faculties at the doctoral degree granting universities spend higher percentages of time on research tasks after accounting for the teaching activity. In higher-level institutions, usually more time is devoted to research. In 1969, the range was from 12 to 35 percent, with the ideal time 45 percent (Parsons & Platt, 1969). Later, Baldridge (1978) reported a range of 5 to 25 percent, with an average time on the task as 14 percent.

Although few empirical studies have been done to determine faculty research time, Lia-Hoagberg (1985) compared college women and nurse doctorates. The percentage of time spent on research and scholarly writing was 26.80 percent for the college women and 16.47 percent for the nurse doctorates. The emphasis placed on research by the institution and the individual faculty's motivation to earn rewards have also affected the amount of time given to research. When more time was spent on teaching, faculty were not found to be better teachers compared to those who also published (Stecklein, 1974).

Behymer and Blackburn (1975) examined variables that would best predict publication output for liberal arts faculty. It was found that tenure and pressure to publish contributed insignificantly to faculty research productivity. High academic rank, interest in research, and the ranking or status of research in the employing institution were the best predictors of publication productivity.

Whether the nursing faculty were productive researchers depended on several conditions (Centra, 1980, p. 34):

- Positive attitude of the dean
- Accepted as role of faculty
- Visible reward systems
- A nonthreatening environment
- Adequate research skills
- Gain of self-rewards
- Available institutional support
- Value of research activity
- Established research mission
- Ongoing research development program
- Release time from teaching

Ketefian (1977) believed that nursing faculty with relatively little research experience could be involved in research and could become productive. Support in terms of budget and staff for nursing research could be found within the school of nursing and throughout the campus, i.e., computer center, grants office, and library.

In 1979, research workload for nursing faculty was ranked third after teaching and service (Fawcett, 1979). A belief existed that the socialization of the new nursing faculty would encourage a role as a productive researcher. Nursing educators did not accept the research responsibility as inherent in the faculty role.

Nursing faculty are beginning to integrate research and scholarly activities into the typical faculty workload. The strategies of integrating research, according to Fawcett (1979), involve priorities for settings (clinical or college), and choice of time. Creativity in ideas and a normal curiosity, in addition to statistical knowledge and computer skills, are beneficial to potential researchers. Replications and cluster studies characteristically are less difficult to initiate. Faculty groups can support one another in mutual collaborative research efforts.

Whatever predicts faculty publication, productivity is a challenging question. Among the many possible variables, current job socialization factors and motivational factors were found to account for at least half of the variance in a study with over 422 full-time tenure-track nursing faculty, teaching in baccalaureate, master's, and doctoral programs (Ostmoe, 1986).

Research as a part of faculty workload in nursing ranked a higher second in priority as an important activity for nursing educators (Henry, 1981). In nursing as in other disciplines, the research workload continues to include grant writing in anticipation of funding intramurally or for extramural support. Following the completion of the projects, the presentation of a scholarly paper before a professional group to disseminate the knowledge of findings is the expectation as well as publishing in journals (Andreoli & Musser, 1984).

With research and scholarly activity, the time spent on workload is more difficult to establish than with teaching productivity. However, the number of publications is concrete documentation. Formulas for quantification of research productivity are more elusive. The assessment of the quality of the research produced again is the most difficult to evaluate.

The production of research will motivate faculty for further scientific inquiry. Faculty will question what nursing is and what should be taught in the curriculum. The continuing research and teaching workload should enhance the quality and outcomes of each.

Service Workload

Service to the university, to the profession, and to the community is an integral part of faculty workload. The service aspect of the faculty workload has been one of the three major workload categories in higher education throughout the years. However, the teaching and research workloads have been more easily identified and measured.

Service has been defined as internal when the activities of the faculty are directed to meeting the goals of the department, the college, or the university. Service is external when the activities are directed to the community or the profession.

Institutional Service. The earlier classifications of faculty service workload were institutional service and public service. Institutional service includes everything from the general administrative responsibilities such as correspondence, telephone conversations, to other conferencing reports or minutes for committee and meetings of all types.

The meetings included a wide range, from departmental subcommittee meetings to university-wide faculty meetings. Attendance at university functions (i.e., commencements, convocations, teas, and receptions) is also included in this category (Yuker, 1974, pp. 20–21).

If the faculty are assigned to specific student service activities (i.e., sponsor for a student organization), the service category is used. An example of an assigned service activity related to students but outside the department is service as student residence advisor. This would also be considered as institutional service.

General administrative functions, serving as departmental chairman, level or program coordinator, associate dean, or dean are considered institutional service. All of the activities that involve student or faculty recruiting, record keeping, budget preparation, public relations, and all communication activities (verbal and written) further expand this category.

Public Service. The terms *public* and *community service* have generally the same meaning. The public service category for faculty service workload includes all professional activities performed outside the institution. Some examples of these are consulting, holding office in a professional organization or editing a professional journal, and giving lectures or speeches to civic groups or to the general public (Yuker, 1974).

Haberman and Quinn (1977, p. 140) listed several criteria for community service activities and a leveling system. Included were service to nonacademic community organizations, i.e., the American Heart Association, and government agencies outside the university, i.e., the state health department. Other contributions of the individual faculty, which could be extended to any community concern are considered service, i.e., voluntary work at health fairs. Any of the activities of the faculty, which would advance the teaching or research mission of the university in the concerns of the community, are faculty service workload.

Levels of Community Service

- **Level one:** lasting over 1 year, extensive consultation, significant program development, coordinating a major research project
- **Level two:** involvement less than a year, assistance with workshops, supervision of projects
- **Level three:** continued service for 2 to 3 months
- **Level four:** one-time activities, few preparation days needed, a public presentation, leading a discussion

For some, leveling of activities has been advantageous in evaluating the time spent by faculty in the service workload (Haberman & Quinn, 1977, p. 140).

Types of Public Service. Dressel (1976) identified three types of public service: national missions, continuing education, and assistance to community groups. The first type was called national missions and followed the agricultural land grant college theme. With federal assistance, the model was extended to business, industry, and urban problems. The second type was continuing education. This category of faculty service workload included the offerings of nondegree courses, workshops, and seminars for professional peers and adults. The third type of public service was assistance to community groups.

The public service workload has been a major professional responsibility for some faculty. It has been evaluated in some institutions and weighted for promotion and tenure decisions (Centra, 1980). Service across disciplines has remained one of the three major missions of the university. The time used for service must directly affect the educational mission of the institution.

Off-campus services are directed as near as the local community, i.e., the neighborhood people who reside in the immediate area of the university. An example would be providing a health promotion fair for the elderly. The state, the nation, and the profession are the large groups served. Included are the state residents and United States citizens as the clients served. In addition, members of professional organizations, the health-related organizations, and the professional peer groups, both within and outside the nursing discipline, are served.

Andreoli (1979) described institutional service for nursing faculty as preparing for, participating in, and writing reports on meetings from the departmental subcommittee meeting to a total all-university setting. Included were commencements, socials, visiting with other nursing schools, and assisting the chairperson or dean with administrative tasks. Public service, according to Andreoli (1979, p. 48), refers to all professional activities (i.e., holding office in a professional organization or participating as a committee member, site visiting, holding office in an organization, which has relevance to the nursing profession, and conducting community health screening or health education programs).

The workload efforts of nursing faculty are major contributions to the university's mission of community service. An example is the establishment of the nursing center or nursing clinic. However, movement in this area has been slow due to the resistance of the physician group (Conway, 1983, p. 15). The recent community nursing center legislation is pending.

Joint collaborative educational projects shared by nursing and other disciplines have offered a broad range of programs serving various groups in the community (i.e., nursery school health supervision, counseling for parents, parenting class preparation for childbirth, and counseling for adolescents) (Conway, 1983, p. 16). Faculty of nursing schools provide a direct service to the community as they work with students in client and family situations. Faculty influence the care of patients and their families and serve as role models for students as part of the laboratory experience (Andruskiw, 1983, p. 30).

Offering consultation to staff of agencies used for clinical placements of nursing students is a visible workload. In a few affiliation agreements between an agency and the school of nursing, a statement is included describing how the faculty will serve on committees or assist in staff development for the agency. Usually faculty are invited to serve on these committees.

Committee work ranked third among the nursing faculty workload factors addressed by Andreoli and Musser (1984). However, public service was ranked fifth following other workload factors of teaching and research.

Service Time. The time spent by faculty in service workload has been estimated to rank third when compared to teaching or research workload. The amount of time devoted to these activities ranged from as low as 8.2 percent (Bayer, 1973) to as high as 21.2 percent (Orlans, 1962).

The average time spent in community service was between 4 and 5 percent of faculty workload in another study. The average time spent in committees and administration was 18 percent of the total workload. Service workload involved less time than undergraduate or graduate teaching or research together. Community service and public service absorbed one-fifth of the faculty workload (Baldridge et al., 1978, p. 102).

Professional Development Workload

A more recent classification of faculty workload has been continuing professional development. While faculty have been expected to remain current in their professional area of expertise, this workload category has been less utilized in higher education throughout the years.

Professional development includes participation by the faculty in various learning activities and some consider practice activities a mechanism of continuing development as a professional. Ideally, practice activities challenge and assist faculty in keeping abreast of current knowledge, skills, and development within their discipline or field of specialization.

The faculty are expected to actively pursue formal study and self-study in the subjects that enable them to maintain high interest, theoretical expertise, and proficiency and competencies of a technical nature. Faculty in nursing have been expected to demonstrate sustained pursuit of lifelong professional learning. The continuous search for learning has provided a stimulus to keep current with issues, trends, and new changes in the practice of professional nursing. Some believe continuous professional development will also stimulate awareness to developments in teaching, in learning methodology for nursing professional development, and research within the nursing discipline.

The activities for nontenured, doctorally prepared faculty and those of the tenured faculty with or without doctoral preparation were found to be similarly goal-oriented. Nondoctorally prepared nontenured faculty would cite the goal of the terminal degree and then document the course work completed toward a degree.

Some of the examples of behaviors or performance of professional development activities for nursing educators include:

- Earning continuing education credits (continuing education unit [CEU])
- Developing proposals for faculty development grants
- Receipt of faculty development grants
- Receipt of a postdoctoral fellowship

- Award of professional certification
- Continuing licensure as a professional nurse
- Documented attendance at professional meetings, workshops, and seminars
- Presentations at faculty collegia

How much professional development is required of the faculty and how much should be classified as part of the faculty workload has been debated within general education. While certain activities may be accepted as professional development, many are not as clearly categorized (i.e., general reading, participating with faculty in discussion, and attending seminars on time or stress management). Theoretically, all outside work of a faculty not specifically assigned could be classified as professional development and not counted as a part of the workload at all (Lorents, 1971, p. 45).

Yuker (1974) presented professional development in a broad definition, which stated it was almost everything that a college professor does. "Everything the faculty does" includes both activities directly related to professional growth and activities only vaguely related. Directly related activities are attending meetings and conventions devoted to scholarly pursuits, taking courses, and participating in faculty discussions on professional topics. Excluded are time spent reading newspapers and magazines, watching television, or engaging in general discussions of nonprofessional topics (Yuker, 1984, p. 22).

The opportunity for professional growth has been a sought-after and desirable consideration for many professionals. Nurses and nurse educators cited professional growth as the most important element in job search (Godfrey, 1975).

The nursing faculty workload analysis of Holliman (1977) found that 5 days out of a total of 225 productive days per academic year are spent by the faculty for professional advancement (i.e., attendance at workshops and conferences). The various other activities considered a part of professional development were not measured. Opportunities in employment for individual professional growth have been strongly identified as desirable by nurses.

Faculty Practice Workload

Andreoli (1979) listed professional development among the activities of the nursing faculty. Andreoli and Musser's (1984) later model of nursing faculty productivity included nursing practice, school administration, and university professional and community service as service workload. The practice component of faculty service included clinical nursing, for which there was responsibility and accountability for the outcome of patient care over and above the supervision of students.

Practice as a type of service included in nursing faculty workload is not widely accepted. If one accepts the challenge for faculty to engage in and maintain practice activities in order to stay proficient in teaching students, then faculty will practice for continuing expertise. An example is the joint appointment. Whether practice is included in the workload will depend on many factors and vary from institution to institution. What is certain is that practice will be an added burden on nursing faculty (Dickens, 1983, p. 121).

Time spent in the direct practice of nursing is included as long as the nurse faculty member is directly responsible for patient care. This category also includes the reading of the nursing literature; attendance at professional meetings, conventions, and workshops; taking courses relevant to nursing; and participating in faculty discussion on professional topics.

Faculty practice has been differentiated as a separate workload category in some institutions (Kent, 1980). However, many believe the practice of the faculty may belong in the professional development category because practice provides active involvement in clinical nursing and maintenance of clinical expertise. Others believe the supervision of students in the clinical area assists faculty in maintaining current practice knowledge and skills.

Professional growth was a category of nursing faculty workload at the University of Iowa (Solomons, Jordison, & Powell, 1980). Of the total faculty workweek of 52.6 hours, time spent for professional growth varied by rank and ranged from 10.4 percent (5.7 hours) for associate and full professors to 17.3 percent (9.2 hours) for assistant professors. Professional growth includes the acquisition and maintenance practice for professional nursing practice.

Whether faculty practice is considered a separate workload or part of professional development, evaluative criteria and measurement mechanisms will be necessary. Time for clinical practice has been viewed as a specific category of the total workload activities of the faculty (Spero, 1980).

If clinical practice joins the traditional workload categories—teaching, research, service, or advising—the time spent for these others will have to be reduced. In the age of retrenchment, faculty may become overburdened by the total expanded workload while attempting to accommodate increased teaching workload. Much depends on how it is arranged.

Advancement and growth possibilities have been considered motivating factors or job satisfiers. They were clearly identified as such by nursing educators (Lenz & Waltz, 1981). Professional development has been a positive type of workload, more desirable than several of the other types (i.e., research or advising). However, the total workload must be defined clearly prior to any analysis or measurement of productivity.

Advising Workload

Academic advising is an important faculty function, which encompasses both academic and career counseling. Advising activities include but are not limited to helping students to plan their programs, clarifying degree requirements, suggesting electives and complementary majors and minors, assisting students in course selection, monitoring student progress toward graduation, suggesting remedial work or tutoring for students with academic difficulties, suggesting possible postgraduate education, and making referrals for further assistance or counseling.

The concept of student service-oriented activities as a faculty workload category has varied greatly in academia throughout the years. Definitions of services have included all types of student services: student advising programs and participation in projects, student activities, and student performances. Letter writing in behalf of students and giving administrative oversight are sometimes considered support for these activities (Lorents, 1971).

The advising category is being used more in workload measurement. In former years, it was considered to be one of the interactions between faculty and students. The types of interactions involved course work during the instructional time as well as counseling or advisement on student curriculum plans and career guidance.

Astin (1977, p. 184) studied student–faculty interactions. Student ratings of student–faculty relations and closeness to faculty were more positively affected by: small institutions, high-cost institutions, student–faculty interaction, academic involvement, living on campus, church-supported institutions, involvement in research, and involvement with honors. Students who did interact more frequently with faculty reported a much higher degree of satisfaction with student–faculty relations then students who did not interact with faculty.

Others have included all interactions with students and with their parents, coaching athletics, or directing any student events as advising workload (Manning & Romney, 1973). Some assigned duties with regard to student registration for courses and special class advising sessions were considered advising workload. The time spent by faculty to update themselves on registration procedures in preparation for the registration process is advisement workload.

Types of Advisement Workload. Advisement workload has been divided into two types: (1) informational advising, and (2) career and personal counseling. Informational advising refers to basic responsibilities of curriculum advice, which consumes 80 percent of the total time for advisement (Kramer & Gardner, 1977). Career and personal counseling fill the remaining 20 percent of the advising workload.

The advising role has tended to be the responsibility of the entire teaching staff. In past years, counseling centers have conducted the student advising sessions. Personal counseling for students has been available from a counseling center.

Some of the basic activities of effective advisement include (Centra, 1980, p. 125):

- Adviser knowledge of curriculum requirements and college policies and procedures: the adviser should know the courses, prerequisites, requirements for the major, credit overload totals, and drop-add procedure.
- Adviser availability: the adviser should keep office hours posted, arrange for extra advising sessions, and willingly take time for advisees.
- Adviser acquaintance with other support services on campus: financial aid and personal counseling.

One reason that advising has become a much more important faculty activity is the present situation of declining student enrollments. In some colleges, advising has become a creative marketing strategy, which may increase and maintain retention rates.

Advising can become a totally individualized and comprehensive program. It is one of the few faculty workload activities other than teaching that provides a purposeful environment for encouraging student–faculty interaction at the undergraduate level.

Advisee Workload. Usually each full-time teaching faculty member is assigned a group of students for advisement. Some faculty are also assigned for the pool of premajor advisers for the college. The advisee assignment has been made by the dean or delegated to another faculty. It can include from 5 or fewer advisees up to 15 or 20 advisees. The number of advisees is determined to yield a compatible workload among the faculty.

Students are preferably assigned to a faculty advisor upon admission to the student's program. Efforts are made to avoid changing the advisee–advisor assignment. However, due to changes in teaching load, changes in research, or faculty turnover, it may become necessary to change the initial assignment.

Student advisee groupings may include various levels of students. Students entering the nursing major as freshmen or sophomores, upper-division generic students, juniors or seniors, and students with previous technical nursing education are best advised by undergraduate faculty. Graduate students potentially make up the graduate faculty's advisement workload.

Advisee workload has been calculated in some universities by means of a standard (i.e., a group of 20 advisees was equal to a 1-credit-hour teaching load). This standard assumed the average faculty member spent two hours per week for each credit hour of teaching. Thus, each advisee would receive approximately an hour and a half per semester toward dedicated advisement (Centra, 1980, p. 126).

Advising Time. The percentage of faculty time devoted to academic advising has varied greatly during the years until the present time. The time spent by faculty on advising workload has differed greatly. The amount of a faculty member's time devoted to student advisement was 12.4 percent (Bayer, 1973).

Some faculty have consumed more time with advisement because they have enjoyed the interaction with students. Others have spent less time engaged in the advisement process, either because they found it less enjoyable or they simply had other more enjoyable work or a workload of higher priority.

Because of the various student class levels, major and premajor advising, and individual advising for courses of study, the role of the advisor has great impact on the student. Accurate direction and guidance of the student throughout the curriculum is imperative and should be emphasized. Unnecessary costs for inappropriate courses and excessive time in programs due to advisement errors can be prevented. Colleges expect quality advisement. In others, advising has been accepted as a vital component of the faculty role, with every faculty member involved in appropriate advising. Guiding and counseling students toward the identification and achievement of graduation has become the advisor's goal.

Advising as nursing faculty workload was in practice for many years. It was identified in the literature by Ketefian (1977) and more recently by Andreoli and Musser (1984). However, performance evaluation criteria for the activities of advisement have not yet been well developed or utilized. The need for both quantitative and qualitative criteria for judging advisement has been recognized. Many collegiate nursing programs have developed guidelines.

ANALYSIS OF FACULTY WORKLOAD

Faculty resources represent the largest expenditure input to the production process in higher education. How the nurse educator as a human resource interfaces with nursing programs demands cost analysis based on workload analysis.

Faculty workload analysis has been considered very important for several other reasons. Such information has been requested by the accreditation agencies and used to assure general efficiency of the instructional programs.

An analysis can be used to develop objective criteria for planning, to determine future loads, or to prevent inequitable loads. Analysis of workload may be utilized for recommending promotion or merit increases for faculty. Faculty workload activity analysis has as its primary use the development of a basis for allocating costs of education.

Humanism and sexism have been explored by workload analysts in education. Nurse educators for the most part have been women. Women have been compared to men in regard to workload productivity. Women in other higher education disciplines have also been compared to nurse educators.

Earlier, in 1975, administrative functions were designated as major activities of nurse doctorates (Pitel & Vian, 1975). It is believed that the shortage of nurse administrators in higher education (i.e., deans, directors, and chairpersons) has reduced the time available for nursing educational administrators to engage in research. Their potential or productivity is reduced for generating new knowledge.

In the study reported in 1983 (Brimmer et al., 1983), nurse educators with doctorates initially hired as instructors changed workload and became engaged in administrative duties. The percentage hired for administration increased to 40 percent in the current position from 22 percent in the first position. Also, the time spent on research decreased from 8 percent in the first position after receiving the doctoral degree to 6 percent for research in their current positions.

When activities of nurse doctorates were compared to other women academics, the findings showed significantly more time was spent on research and more journal articles were published by the non-nurse group. Although teaching remained the primary function for both groups, nurses with doctorates spent more time in administrative activities (Lia-Hoagberg, 1985).

The problem of documenting actual workload activities has been well established. Self-reporting by faculty on their work activities has not been considered to be reliable. Laughlin and Lestrad (1976) reported that activity analysis was difficult for faculty to assess due to pressures of declining enrollment, tenure insecurity, student evaluations, and increased productivity expectations.

A study in 1978 revealed a high degree of similarity in faculty workload activity data between assigned (chairperson reporting) and reported (faculty self-reporting data) (Coleman & Peeples, 1978). But faculty has reported less time spent on instructional activity than was assigned in another study. More time was reported by faculty as spent on noninstructional activities. If this analysis were utilized to generate a program budget, instructional costs would become decreased and costs for community service, for example, could be increased (Laughlin & Lestrad, 1976).

Faculty workload data can be difficult to discern from department to department. It has been a problem for an outsider to a given specialty department to determine if an individual faculty load in one department is significantly greater or less than in another (Conway, 1983, p. 93).

The analysis of faculty workload was an issue predicted to be related to public and private appropriations in the 1980s (Henard, 1979). Performance budgets, performance audits, and program evaluations have become integrally related to faculty workload. As higher education becomes dedicated to an input–output (resources–product) orientation, workloads of faculty have been more scrutinized. Productivity audits of faculty activities can be utilized to derive and realign program budgets. Reduction in the number of faculty through increasing faculty workload has resulted.

What needs to be accomplished for each college nursing department is a total analysis of all workload activities by faculty and the actual time spent on the activity. The resulting faculty activity analysis could become the tool utilized for establishing weighted formulas and productivity measures.

In 1983, a survey was made of 248 nurse educators to determine the elements of faculty workload. A questionnaire was sent to faculty from programs with memberships in the American Association of Colleges of Nursing (AACN). The results were reported at the annual meeting of the Society for Research in Nursing Education.

The activities or faculty workload elements were ranked by the participants with respect to influence on tenure, promotions, and reappointment decisions (TPR). The percent of time faculty spent engaged in the activity was indicated in Table 5–1 (Zanecchia, 1985).

TABLE 5–1. RANKING OF MEANS: MOST IMPORTANT FACULTY WORKLOAD ELEMENTS TO INFLUENCE TPR DECISIONS

Ranking	Workload Elements	Mean	Percent Time
1.	Teaching	1.96	60.1
2.	Other	2.25	5.9
3.	Research or scholarly presentation	2.43	7.6
4.	Publications	2.75	5.6
5.	Advising	3.21	7.5
6.	Grant writing	3.31	5.6
7.	Administration	3.40	10.4
8.	Continuing education (others)	3.46	3.4
9.	Curriculum	3.58	8.7
10.	Service (on campus)	3.60	6.0
11.	Professional practice	3.63	7.0
12.	Continuing education (self)	3.73	4.2
13.	Consultation	4.03	3.7
14.	Service (off-campus)	4.11	5.0

Number of nurse educators in study = 248.

The other category which consumed approximately 6 percent (3 hours) of the total faculty workweek (50 hours) was identified as time for doctoral preparation. Whether the pursuit of the doctorate is an acceptable element of the faculty workload has been questioned. Some have believed the terminal degree should be pursued in the time outside the faculty workload.

The five highest faculty workload elements found most important for TPR were the major activities of teaching, other research, publications, and advising. Service (on-campus) was ranked tenth, and service (off-campus) was last of 14 activities.

WORKLOAD FORMULAS

Developing useful workload formulas for each nursing faculty in the department is a desirable goal for the individual and the department.

Workload formulas are the mechanisms for planning curriculum, learning objectives, projecting instructor needs, measuring productivity, and evaluating the activities in the workload.

Most time and increased weight is placed on the teaching activity. Service, research, and advising activities of differing weights are usually found in the most typical workload formula.

The individual typical workload formula in faculty productivity units* is

$$FP = T + R + S + A + O$$

where:

T = teaching   60%
R = research   14%
S = service   11%
A = advising   8%
O = other   6%

Departmental faculty workload formulas set guidelines for the activities of a group of faculty in an academic department. Based on the departmental mission and goals, the departmental formula is the compilation of multiple aggregate faculty workload activities. Departmental formulas may and do reflect a variety of weighted workload elements simultaneously.

No two elements need be weighted alike. Formulas may change from year to year. Different workload elements may be included having different weights. For example, a faculty member who has earned a grant to conduct research may have the research activity weighted more heavily in a given formula and the teaching

---

*The definition of a unit is a measure of workload, a percent of time on task, a weight of magnitude prescribed, the number of contact hours.

activity weighted less. A balance must be maintained between the weighted faculty activities to accommodate the various needs of the individual faculty (i.e., research workload and the department or teaching workload).

The workload formulas should be individualized and unique to a specific program. All of the faculty activities, which are viewed as part of the complex faculty role, should be reflected in the total weighted formula. Cost-effectiveness, flexibility, and fairness should describe the formula, which is realistic.

The weighted workload formula method for analyzing faculty productivity has been attempted by many. Determining workable formulas, an acceptable standard work unit, weights, or an equitable adjustment factor have been suggested.

But there has been no uniform plan for implementation. Each individual program and college has developed and used its own established formula, if it has one. Institutions have accepted one or another type of formula according to how faculty salaries are appropriated and how the instructional budgets are generated.

Student outcomes or products have been utilized to predict faculty and program productivity and projected workload formulas. Faculty outputs (research, grants, and publications) were described in Chapter 1 as productive in the Interacting System Model (ISM).

Gulko's (1971) study was a methodological study defining unit costs in the educational environment. A major portion of the study described the algebra of unit costs. The algebra provided a mathematical relationship between the variables of discipline, course level, direct cost, number of students, total cost, average cost, and FTE student cost.

The study also considered indirect costs. The cost per degree awarded consisted of three types of costs: (1) direct instructional cost incurred in generating the degree; (2) the allocated support costs associated with the direct instructional costs; and (3) indirect student support costs generated by virtue of the degree winner being present in the system. Gulko further discussed some of the problems of handling the costs of attrition (no degree awarded), transfer students, both in and out, and transfers between programs.

The workload profile contributed by Holliman (1977) was useful in determining teaching responsibilities for the individual nursing faculty. Teaching was based on the computation of the number of hours available. Classroom teaching, clinical supervision, and preparation time were included. The profile count of the hours required for the same three activities were compared. A differential of being either underutilized or overextended was calculated for each of the faculty. The type of workload analysis when implemented would serve to project workload hours needed. Modifications and redistributions of faculty workload could be considered. Other options were hiring more faculty or changing the curriculum.

In the same year, the work of Tate (1977) proposed a model for determining faculty workload in schools of nursing (shown in Table 5–2). A similar dyad was described. Faculty workload was perceived as having the dimensions of time spent on actual teaching of lecture and laboratory and time required for preparation, student evaluation, and counseling. These were described as contact hour and noncontact hour workload.

TABLE 5–2. TATE FACULTY WORKLOAD MODEL

$$1 \text{ contact class hour} = 1 \text{ TWH}_c{}^a$$
$$\frac{NS^c (NLh)^d}{8} = \text{TWH}_{Lh}{}^b$$
$$\text{TWH}_c + \text{TWH}_{Lh} = \text{TWH}^e$$
$$12 \text{ to } 14 \text{ TWH} = 1 \text{ FTW}^f$$

[a] Teacher workload hour for class contact time
[b] Teacher workload hour for laboratory contact time
[c] Number of students for laboratory
[d] Number of laboratory contact hours
[e] Teacher workload hours
[f] Full-time teacher workload

The model presented was based on contact hours. Eight was the denominator in the equation for determining teacher workload hours of laboratory, with the mean recommended 1:8 for the teacher–student ratio.

The University of Wisconsin Milwaukee School of Nursing developed guidelines for faculty workload. The faculty recognized that the determination of workload was the responsibility of the academic department or program unit. The faculty established 40 units as the standard workload for the semester. But it did not equate units with the 35 to 45 hours of time spent working in the average workweek.

The three major functions of the faculty—teaching, service, and research—were analyzed. Suggested equivalencies for various activities were determined. For example, an undergraduate lecture hour for over 25 students was 5 units, while the same hour was 3 units when students numbered under 25.

Graduate lecture or seminar hours were equivalent to 3 units if attended by ten or fewer students. The same seminar yielded 5 units if more than ten students attended. Undergraduate laboratory hours were each equivalent to 1 unit. A graduate practicum hour had 2.5 units.

Service as a chairperson of ten faculty or less earned 10 units, while over ten faculty yielded 20 units. Activity as the chairperson of a department committee was 1 unit for every 5 hours of meetings. The university committee chairperson assignment earned 20 units. Memberships of department and university committees were equivalent to 1 unit for 10 hours of meetings and 10 units, respectively.

Research activities were equivalent to 10 units. Grants for other support for the research could result in up to 40 equivalent units (Saylor, Kaylor, Genthe, & Otis, 1979). Many of the activities of the faculty were not included in the guidelines, but the tool was found to be useful.

WORKLOAD BALANCE AND WEIGHTING

Many factors must be determined to assess or analyze the workload of nursing faculty. The multiple role and responsibilities have demanded that faculty members: be excellent teachers, have a doctorate, be clinical models, practice nursing, keep current in knowledge, be active in research, be agency liaisons, innovate curriculum, be active in organizations, participate on committees, and develop themselves professionally. Wardle (1984) asked where these workload activities would end.

Nursing education, as nursing service, is labor intensive. The major costs of higher education are derived from staffing the faculty. The workload activities of the faculty become the staffing costs of the nursing educational program.

In earlier years, Plawecki and Plawecki (1976) had written that the workload of nurse faculty was an important recruitment and retention factor for nurse educators. Others stated that the work satisfaction of nursing educators was important. Retention of faculty was attributed to supportive colleagues, keeping current, and having autonomy (Grandjean, Aiken, & Bonjean, 1976). Higher turnover rates have been considered to be more costly. Assessing faculty specialties as staffing resources must be completed prior to balancing and weighting workload. The strategy of workload balance through weighting the workload activities is in its infancy. Formula-driven workload analysis creates a need to monitor nursing faculty activities more carefully as they attempt to do all and be all.

Various weighted workload formulas exist throughout collegiate nursing education. Formulas with differing workload units have been defined and utilized by individual college nursing programs. It is unlikely that a universal workload formula could be developed that would be suitable for all programs. If so, an average workload could consist of 40 work units per week. For example, faculty could be assigned a teaching load of not less than 6 or more than 9 course credit hours per semester, as shown in Table 5–3. Units for scholarly or service activities might consist of a unit for each clock hour of: proposal development; research; professional writing; presentation at professional meetings and preparation and consultation; school, university, professional, and community service; and professional practice.

Another type of load formula may differentiate teaching load in the classroom for junior-level classes (2.8 credit hours per week) from senior level with 3 credit hours per week. Clinical teaching loads vary in some institutions from a load of 7.5 credit hours to 9 credit hours. (One credit hour may be equal to 2 contact hours.) Time distribution for a typical faculty workweek might consist of the following workload breakdown based on a 55-hour week (Table 5–4):

While most workload formulas for classroom teaching utilize 1 credit hour as

TABLE 5–3. COLLEGE WORKLOAD UNIT

- 4 units for each course clock hour
- 1.5 units for each clinical clock hour
- 1.5 units for each laboratory clock hour
- 2 units for each thesis committee clock hour as chairman
- 1 unit for each thesis committee clock hour as member
- 1 unit for each advising or counseling clock hour

TABLE 5-4. WEEKLY WORKLOAD DISTRIBUTION

Type	Credit Hours	Preparation Hours	Contact Hours
Teaching	12	—	—
Lecture	—	6	3
Clinical	—	16	15
Advising	—	—	4
Service	—	—	6
Research	—	—	5
Total	12	22	33

equal to 1 load unit, some institutions accept .5 or .66 credits per 1 clinical contact hour. Other variations can depend on the number of students enrolled. When more than ten students are enrolled, the load credit is calculated from the number of students. The load credit is increased .5 for every ten additional students. A faculty load plan based on a 60-hour week semester with 4 hours per week equals to 1 load credit (Table 5-5).

Attempts have been made to equalize the nursing faculty workload and to comparatively weight the different types of activities in which faculty engage. The demands made on the faculty's time in classroom teaching versus clinical teaching has been a controversial issue (Crawford et al, 1983, p. 285).

A weighted formula devised at the University of Saskatchewan was based on two separate factors for preparation time. Two hours of preparation time were allowed for each hour of lecture. One hour of preparation time was allowed for each 3 hours of clinical teaching.

TABLE 5-5. TYPICAL FACULTY WORKLOAD GUIDELINES FOR A 60-HOUR WEEK

Percent Time	Activity	Hours per Week	Units
44	Teaching		
	6 graduate credits	24	6.0
	9 undergraduate credits	36	9.0
5	Advising 15 advisees at .03 units	2	0.5
1	Committees	4	0.23
10	Research	4	1.0
10	Administration	2	1.0
10	Service	4	1.0
10	Continuing education	4	1.0
10	Practice	4	1.0
100		60	15.0

One load credit equals 4 hours per week or 60 hours per semester.

Faculty Teaching Workload Formula

$$\left[\frac{a + 2a + b + \frac{b}{3}}{c} \right] d = x \text{ units}$$

where:

a = Number of hours of lecture and seminar per week
$2a$ = Preparation time for lecture and seminar
b = Number of hours of clinical and laboratory per week
$\frac{b}{3}$ = Preparation time for clinical and laboratory
c = Average weekly teaching load and preparation for the university as a whole
d = Number of weeks in term
x = Number of units for teaching load

The normal teaching load for an academic year has been determined to be 26 units. The teaching load for the semester is 9.88 units. If the assumption that three fifths of the total load is teaching, then the overall workload is 42 units. The remaining units would be divided between research or practice of professional skill (10 units) and committee work, administration, and college and public service (6 units).

A unit for research is equal to 27 hours. Every full-time tenure-track faculty has the equivalent of 270 hours or 7 weeks of time available for research and practice. 10 hours of meeting time is equivalent to 1 unit, with a chairmanship doubling the unit value. Service weightings range from .5 units to 1 unit for activities (i.e., planning committee for nursing continuing education, presentation of workshops, professional lectures to a community group, and participation in professional organizations).

Each program and college that designs an individualized equitable algorithm for determining faculty load will affect productivity. Although academicians have reported 40- to 60-hour workweeks including two thirds of time on teaching, research, and service, other professionals also spend as much time.

Faculty who teach 30 credit hours per academic year have 1 scheduled lecture hour per week per semester, equaling 1 instructor credit hour. 3 scheduled laboratory hours per week per semester equals 2 instructor credit hours, and 3 scheduled hours per week per semester of academic conferences equals 2 instructor credit hours. 6 scheduled nursing clinical hospital laboratory hours per week per semester equals 5 instructor credit hours (Goeres, 1978). Whichever workload standard is selected, it should be equally weighted and operationalized.

PRODUCTIVITY AND WORKLOAD STRATEGIES

The implementation of strategies to control, change, or reduce workload formulas has been a necessary task. With the current economic situation, nursing faculty workload cannot be reduced by hiring more faculty. However, three other strategies were suggested by Dienemann (1983):

- Diversification of income
- Structure and modes of teaching
- Faculty mix

Grants, alumni contributions, and fees for client services from faculty and students will increase revenues. These and changing teaching methodologies could affect workload for faculty (i.e., increases in class sizes). Utilization of teaching assistants was a strategy also suggested by Dienemann.

More extensive utilization of master's-prepared preceptors would alleviate some strain on the teaching faculty resources. Delegation of clinical teaching to assistants (i.e., teaching assistants or T.A.s) and grading papers would free up some faculty time for the other workload activities of research or service.

Timing Strategy

When workload formulas have been weighted, the timing of workload becomes important. In a given year, the activities of greater weight are priorities for the department and the individual faculty. Individual faculty could share load with teaching team members with benefit to all. Level teams could share load and implement a timing strategy for assignments.

Plans for execution of funded research grants or the implementation of a special project such as new or revised curriculum can be generated in advance of the activity. Faculty teaching loads, which are modified to meet 5-year workload plans are lighter in a research grant year.

Faculty have been given "released" time from normal teaching loads to accommodate other service, scholarly activities, or professional continuing education and study in their area of expertise. Faculty productivity in the practice role has been enhanced by allowing faculty an open quarter, approximately 10 weeks, during the year. Other activities in which faculty could participate include reading for manuscript development, presentations at professional meetings consultation, or designing innovative curriculum modalities (Gay, 1984).

The creative scheduling of time for teaching classes and clinical laboratories can usually provide faculty one day per week for scholarly work. Timing arrangements in the teaching schedule can reduce one faculty workload and double another. Faculty have alternated times for lighter and double workload assignments.

Faculty Mix Strategy

A faculty group with an adequate mix of types and numbers will enhance productivity. Ratios of full-time to part-time are best established by the individual program. Although part-time faculty do cost less, having a lower salary and few benefits, the negative perspective is their lack of mastery of the college mission and academic policies (Lane, 1983). Also, they lack input into curriculum and clinical implementation, evaluation, advising, and research.

Other elements of faculty mix are available, and no best mix exists. The need for faculty resources and productivity should determine mix. Faculty mix elements include: full-time to part-time, tenured to nontenured, flexible-course to specific-course-only assignment, higher faculty ranks to lower faculty ranks, theory lecture teaching to clinical laboratory teaching, doctorates to nondoctorates, grant producers to nongrant producers, retiring to nonretiring, retention to nonretention, and regularly appointed to visiting adjunct and joint appointments.

Collaborative Strategy

Collaborative strategies have been suggested as a method for increasing nursing faculty productivity. Joint appointments of faculty have been made. Education and practice workload has been concurrently assigned.

Many believe collaborative arrangement will partially solve the ongoing dilemma for the nurse educator, which was described as a lack of clinical expertise. Some of the other models included dual appointments, private practice, development of a practice within a nursing college, and assuming care for patients while supervising students (Kruger, 1985).

Interdisciplinary collaboration to support teaching workload in the nursing department may increase productivity. Non-nurse faculty teaching non-nursing courses (i.e., statistics, nutrition, physiology, pathophysiology, or research methods) could free nursing faculty for more research (Lenz, 1985).

The input–output interacting system model provides a basis for measuring productivity. The needs and skills of the individual faculty must be integrated with the goals and objectives of the institution. The demands placed upon the faculty must be balanced with the nature of the tasks that make up the workload. The entire work environment must also be considered. Productivity for the nurse educator depends upon the comprehensive planned interaction of these many elements.

REFERENCES

Abdellah, F. G., & Levine, E. (1965). *Better patient care through nursing research.* New York: Macmillan.
Andreoli, K. G. (1979). Faculty productivity. *Journal of Nursing Administration, 9*(11), 47–53.
Andreoli, K. G., & Musser, L. A. (1984). Improving nursing faculty productivity. *Nurse Educator, 9*(2), 9–15.
Andruskiw, O. (1983). A socio-humanistic model of administration. In M. E. Conway and O. Andruskiw, *Administrative theory: Issues in and higher education in nursing practice: Issues in higher education in nursing,* (p. 1930). E. Norwalk, Conn.: Appleton-Century-Crofts.
Astin, A. (1977). *Four critical years* (pp. 184–186). San Francisco: Jossey-Bass Publishers.
Baldridge, J. V.; Curtis, D. V.; Ecker, G. E.; & Riley, G. L. (1978). *Policy making and effective leadership* (p. 102). San Francisco: Jossey-Bass Publishers.
Bayer, A. E. (1973). Teaching faculty in academe: 1972–1973. *ACE Research Reports, 8,* 1–68.

Behymer, C. E., & Blackburn, R. T. (1975). *Environmental and personal attributes related to faculty productivity.* (Arlington, Va.: Eric Document No. ED 104317)
Bogue, F. G. (1972). Method and meaning in faculty activity analysis. In C. T. Stewart (Ed.), *Reformation and reallocation in higher education.* 12th Annual Forum of the Association for Institutional Research. Claremont, Calif.: Association for Institutional Research.
Bowen, H. R. (1977). *Investment in learning: The individual and social value of American higher education* (p. 11). San Francisco: Jossey-Bass Publishers.
Brimmer, P. F.; Skoner, M. M.; Pender, N. J.; Williams, C. A.; Fleming, J. W.; & Werley, H. H. (1983). Nurses with doctoral degrees: Educational and employment characteristics (p. 157–165). *Research in Nursing and Health, 6.*
Centra, J. (1980). *Determining faculty effectiveness* (p. 34). San Francisco: Jossey-Bass Publishers.
Coleman, D. R., & Peeples, T. O. (1978). Faculty activity assignment versus faculty effort. Paper presented at the 11th Annual Florida Statewide Conference on Institutional Research, Orlando, Florida.
Conway, M. E. (1983). The professional school in the university. In M. E. Conway and O. Andruskiw, *Administrative theory and practice: Issues in higher education in nursing* (pp. 81–99). E. Norwalk, Conn.: Appleton-Century-Crofts.
Crawford, M. E.; Laing, G.; Linwood, M.; Kyle, M.; & DeBlock, A. (1983). A formula for calculating faculty workload. *Journal of Nursing Education, 22*(7), 285–286.
Dickens, M. (1983). Faculty practice and social support. *Nursing Leadership, 6*(4), 121–128.
Dienemann, J. (1983). Reducing nursing faculty workloads without increasing costs. *Image, 15*(4), 111–114.
Dressel, P. L. (1976). *Handbook of academic evaluation: Assessing institutional effectiveness, student progress and professional performance for decision making in higher education.* San Francisco: Jossey-Bass Publishers.
Fawcett, J. (1979, April 27). Integrating research into the faculty workload. *Nursing Outlook,* 259–262.
Gay, J. T. (1984). Faculty release quarter time. *Nursing and Health Care, 5*(1), 37–39.
Godfrey, M. (1975). Your fringe benefits: How much are they really worth? *Nursing, 75*(5), 73–75.
Goeres, E. R. (1978). Faculty productivity. *Collective Bargaining Perspectives, 3*(5), 3.
Grandjean, B. D.; Aiken, L. H.; & Bonjean, C. M. (1976). Professional autonomy and the work satisfaction of nursing educators. *Nursing Research, 25* 216–221.
Gulko, W. W. (1971). *The research requirements prediction model (RRPM-1): An overview.* Boulder, Colo.: Western Interstate Commission for Higher Education, 29.
Haberman, M., & Quinn, L. (1977). Assessing faculty's community service. *Adult Leadership, 25,* 140–150.
Henard, R. E. (1979, May). The impacts of the faculty workload emphasis on postsecondary education in the 1980s (p. 17). Paper presented at the 19th Annual Forum of the Association for Institutional Research, San Diego, California.
Henderson, A. D., & Henderson, J. G. (1974). *Higher education in America* (pp. 148–152). San Francisco: Jossey-Bass Publishers.
Henry, J. K. (1981). Nursing and tenure. *Nursing Outlook, 29*(4), 240–244.
Holliman, J. M. (1977). Analyzing faculty workload. *Nursing Outlook, 25,* 721–723.
Holzemer, W. L. (1982). Quality in graduate nursing education. *Nursing Health Care, 3*(10), 536–542.

Kent, N. A. (1980). Evaluating the practice component for faculty rank and tenure. *Cognitive Dissonance: Interpreting and Implementing Faculty Practice Roles in Nursing Education* (pp. 21–25). New York: National League for Nursing.
Ketefian, S. (1977). An exchange research experience. *Nursing Outlook, 25,* 454–56.
Koos, L. V. (1919). *The adjustment of the teaching load in a university* (p. 5) (Dept. of the Interior, Bureau of Education, Bulletin No. 15 271–272). Washington, D.C.: Government Printing Office.
Kramer, H. C., & Gardner, R. E. (1977). *Advising by faculty.* Washington, D.C.: National Education Association.
Kruger, H. C. (1985). The demonstration of a joint faculty/practice position. *Journal of Nursing Education, 24*(8), 350–352.
Lane, J. A. (1983, October). Tactical practices for maintaining the integrity of nursing program: The private sector. Paper given at the American Association of Colleges of Nursing, Colorado Springs, Colorado.
Laughlin, J. S., & Lestrad, V. A. (1976). Faculty load and faculty activity analysis: Who considers the individual faculty member? Proceedings of the 16th Annual Forum of the Association for Institutional Research. Los Angeles, California.
Lenz, E. R. (1985). Disciplinary boundary maintenance in nursing education. *Journal of Nursing Education, 24*(8), 325–331.
Lenz, E. R., & Waltz, C. F. (1981, December). *Relations of demographic characteristics, work environment and job search activities in job satisfaction of nursing educators in the south.* Presented at the First Southern Council for Collegiate Education in Nursing Research.
Lia-Hoagberg, B. (1985). Comparison of professional activities of nurse doctorates and other women academics. *Nursing Research, 34*(3), 155–159.
Lorents, A. C. (1971). *Faculty activity analysis and planning models in higher education.* St. Paul, Minn.: Higher Education Coordinating Commission. (ED055571)
Manning, C. W., & Romney, L. C. (1973). *Faculty activity analysis: Procedures manual.* Boulder, Colo.: Western Interstate Commission for Higher Education. (HE004891)
Marsh, H. W. (1979, June). Total faculty earnings, academic productivity and demographic variables. Paper presented at the Annual Academic Planning Conference. Los Angeles: University of Southern California Office of Institutional Studies. (ED181819)
Minter, W. J., & Bowen, H. R. (1982, May 19). Colleges' achievements in recent years came out of the hides of professors. *The Chronicle of Higher Education,* 8.
Moos, R. (1979). *Evaluating educational environments: Procedures, measures, findings and policy implications.* San Francisco: Jossey-Bass Publishers.
Murphy, J. F. (1978, March). Tenure: Achieved or ascribed. *Nursing Outlook,* 176–179.
Orlans, H. (1962). *The effects of federal programs on higher education.* Washington, D.C.: Brookings Institution.
Ostmoe, P. M. (1986). Correlates of university nurse faculty publication productivity. *Journal of Nursing Education, 25*(15), 209–212.
Pace, C. R. (1979). *Measuring outcomes of college.* San Francisco: Jossey-Bass Publishers.
Parsons, T., & Platt, G. M. (1969). *The American academic profession, a research proposal.* Submitted to the National Science Foundation. Cambridge, Mass.: Harvard University.
Pitel, M., & Vian, J. (1975). Analysis of nurse doctorates. *Nursing Research, 24,* 340–351.
Plawecki, J. A., & Plawecki, H. M. (1976). Factors that influence attraction and retention of qualified nurse educators. *Nursing Research, 25,* 133–135.

Saylor, A. A.; Kaylor, L. E.; Genthe, D.; & Otis, E. (1979). Guidelines for faculty workload. *American Journal of Nursing, 79*(5), 902–904.

Shils, E. (1972). Intellectuals, tradition and the tradition of intellectuals: Some preliminary considerations. *Daedalus, 101,* 21–34.

Solomons, H. C.; Jordison, N. S.; & Powel, S. R. (1980). How faculty members spend their time. *Nursing Outlook, 28*(3), 160–165.

Spero, J. (1980). A professional practice discipline in academia. *Nursing and Health Care, 1*(21), 22–25.

Stecklein, J. E. (1974). Approaches to measuring workload over the past two decades. In J. E. Doi (Ed.), *Assessing faculty effort* (pp. 1–16). San Francisco: Jossey-Bass Publishers.

Stickler, W. H. (1960). Working material and bibliography on faculty load. In K. Bunnell (Ed.), *Faculty workload* (pp. 80–97). Washington, D.C.: American Council on Education.

Tate, E. T. (1977). A model for determining faculty workload in schools of nursing (p. 5). Dissertation Summary No. 86. Baton Rouge: Louisiana State University.

Templin, J. L. (1983). Productivity and the supervisor. *The Health Care Supervisor, 1*(3), 1–11.

Wardle, M. G. (1984, Summer). How does one get it all done? *Nurse Educator, 9*(2), 16–17.

Young, L. C. (1985). *Dimensions of professional nursing.* New York: Macmillan.

Yuker, H. E. (1974). *Faculty workload: Facts, myths, and commentary* (p. 20). (Report No. 6, American Association for the Study of Higher Education). Washington, D.C.: The George Washington University.

Yuker, H. E. (1984). *Faculty workload: Research, theory, and interpretation.* (p. 10). (Report No. 10, American Association for the Study of Higher Education). Washington, D.C.: The George Washington University.

Zanecchia, M. D. (1981). A study of the relationships of nursing faculty productivity, nursing student attributes and outcomes (Doctoral dissertation, University of Connecticut, 1981). *Dissertation Abstracts International, 42,* 4B.

Zanecchia, M. D. (1985, January). Faculty workload elements and forces affecting nursing education. *Proceedings and Abstracts* (pp. 18–20). 3rd Annual Meeting, Research in Nursing Education, Society for Research in Nursing Education, San Francisco.

6

Career Entry

Margaret Denise Zanecchia, Ph.D., R.N.

The quality of nursing education programs has been the concern of many groups in the past, as it is now. Quality continues to be of strong interest for students, health care consumers, nursing educators, nursing service personnel, physicians, hospital administrators, and university administrators. These groups can act as forces, and when their views differ, the control of career entry for nurse educators can become a major challenge to the nursing profession (Brown & Chinn, 1982, p. 66).

Academic leaders have reported increasing difficulty in maintaining a high quality of graduate faculties in sufficient numbers to sustain undergraduate and graduate education (Brademas, 1983, p. 27). In most higher education programs, women have constituted one half of the graduate students and one third of the doctoral students in recent years.

In recent decades, the nursing education system has been given the task of providing an ongoing pool of highly qualified faculty to carry out the instructional mission of the nursing profession. The number of nurses earning doctoral degrees is steadily increasing. Career nurse educators are necessary and needed for all collegiate nursing programs, baccalaureate, master's, and doctoral. Career planning and career development in nursing became more emphasized in the 1970s and 1980s, although in the 1980s, the establishment of specific career goals for the nurse educator gained more attention.

The nursing profession has addressed careers and change in career goals. The importance of educational mobility for individuals wishing to advance from one level of nursing practice to another has been documented by the National League for Nursing (NLN) (1982a). The NLN has offered a position statement that has expressed the requirements for the preparation of the faculty to be a degree in nursing at the master's level and preferably at the doctoral level (National League for Nursing, 1981).

111

Nursing faculty are seeking career education that guarantees greater career mobility and flexibility and that will prepare them for the complexities of the educational environment. Ensuring professional growth and mobility is essential in the recruitment of the most qualified and talented nurse educators (Flanagan, 1981, pp. 15, 29–30).

Career entry development for nurse educators is obtained in many ways. Prior to entry, certain requirements must be met. Formal education for the master's degree is a minimum requirement. Other more informal activities may also take place: continuing education, conferences, workshops, short courses, or attendance at credit-free offerings. Some specific workshops are offered to help potential faculty understand the many aspects of the academic role, including how to develop an individual plan to meet tenure and promotion requirements (National League for Nursing, 1985b).

Nurse educators will need to develop more research and computer skills for a constantly changing and competitive marketplace. The anticipated oversupply of between 20,000 and 70,000 physicians by 1990 will affect nursing and nursing education (White, 1983). Physicians may assume former roles of nurse specialists. Since costs for physician services outweigh those of nursing, the physician glut could be an advantage for nursing (Kelly, 1985; Andreoli & Musser, 1985).

Career pathways for the nurse educator in the college systems may be influenced by the effects of the physician surplus. Specialists in nursing may seek employment in academia if physicians reclaim these expanded practice roles once given to them.

The nurse educator prepares nurses as generalists and for specialization in the college setting. Perceived as an artist, the nurse educator conveys the artistry of nursing to students of professional nursing. According to Butterfield, education involves demonstrating to students how to use resources for gaining new knowledge and implementing research. Education also involves validation of practice so that it will be improved. The knowledge that is gained should be shared (Butterfield, 1985, p. 102).

Career is defined as a profession that trains and that is undertaken as a permanent calling. In the past, a career in nursing was the decision to become a trained nurse. A career in nursing education occurred by being promoted, having seniority, or somehow advancing in the employment setting. Historically, a nurse applied clinical skills at the bedside before progressing to other career alternatives (Ehrat, 1981).

Bolles (1980, p. 100) described a career as a flexible combination of skills, which could be arranged in a number of different and tantalizing ways. The contemporary definition of a career in nursing education encompasses the exercise of selected individualized activities. Career planning is a progression of steps toward a specific faculty position in a college or university setting.

Schwirian (1981, p. 248) identified nursing career behaviors in a model of nursing performance. These behaviors included many goal-directed career nursing education activities that could lead the nurse to a position as a nurse educator. Postgraduate education, professional activities, satisfaction, job performance, and interagency mobility were identified in an open system model. In the Interacting System Model (ISM), many of these same activities, education, and experience are the input or structure of the individual nurse educator who is assessing career entry.

CAREER PLANNING

Entry into any career requires short- and long-range planning. Planning for career entry in other professions has existed for a longer time and is more often documented than career planning in nursing. The benefits of career planning, both personal and professional, are even more important in nursing (Nowak & Grindel, 1984, p. 4). Although nursing is predominantly a woman's profession, the opportunity to exercise control over life-style and significant events is very desirable for both men and women who provide major financial support through employment.

With the newer concept in higher education being "education for all" rather than for a select few, educational career planning is vital for all professionals (Conway & Andruskiw, 1983). Contemporary planning in nursing education includes the planning for career entry as a nurse educator. Even more strategic to the planning are job market analyses for nurse educators and the review of occupational data.

Career planning involves the assessment of self, the individual's structure, and the assessment of the career structure. Although scanty, information on nursing careers has appeared in the literature in recent years; however, topics focused on a career as a nurse educator were even more scarce (Shane, 1983; Anastas, 1984).

The simplest definition of a nursing career development program for nurse educators was adapted from Keough (1977). Career development is an organized system in which goals are set, needs being identified. Counseling and guidance are made available. Plans are implemented and activities are evaluated in order to revise plans as needed.

Varieties of collaborative experiences that blend with a concurrent educational pursuit can be staged at different times in the total life plan. The optimum career development program would provide the long-range concepts that the nurse educator could apply in seeking positions or changing a career. Positions in any college or university setting could be considered, or a career transition outside the nursing discipline.

INDIVIDUAL NURSE EDUCATOR SYSTEM

Entry into the career as a nurse educator first requires an individual structure. The structure in the ISM is defined as the educational degree, experiences (nursing, communication, teaching–learning, and research), and personal goals and values of the nurse.

The individual nurse is the fundamental cell structure, the input of the open system. At any time entry into the nursing educational system occurs, the initial interaction involves the individual educator particularized by prior education and professional and personal life experiences.

Education prerequisites of the system, which are necessary at entry are the appropriate educational degree and preparation for teaching. The degree of choice for the career nurse educator is the master of science in nursing, with the doctorate in nursing as a part of the future plan.

Education

The ISM assumes that four significant internal processes characterize the education of the individual nurse. These processes are:

- Nursing
- Communication
- Teaching–learning
- Research

Nursing Process. The nurse educator's mastery of the fundamental components of the nursing process is necessary. The nursing process parallels the problem-solving process. It is a vital tool for the nurse educator who plans, directs, implements, or evaluates nursing care or modifies the type of instruction that may best facilitate learning.

The nurse educator's application is enhanced with documentation of certification in a nursing specialty with the nursing master's degree, which establishes mastery. Current experiences with the newer technologies will also have a positive influence for the applicant.

Communication Process. The communication process for a nurse educator is another vital function. Effective verbal and writing skills appropriate for various levels of students, peers, and administrators are essential. Consistent communicating with staff in the clinical agency is required at all levels. Computers have and will define the state-of-the-art uses for more sophisticated communication, both in-house or via satellites. Clinical and statistical data will assist the nurse educator to teach students how to implement advanced care techniques in the care of clients. The nurse educator will network, store, retrieve, and extrapolate the most up-to-date health information.

Teaching–Learning Process. The ISM merges two basic approaches in education: the teaching process and the learning process. Education in nursing has been strategically integrated in a complex open system of general education for many decades. The role of the nurse has always included the functions and responsibilities of a teacher. In fact, all nurses have been formally introduced to selected curricular offerings designed to facilitate client education or health-related problems. As an educator, the nurse facilitates the learning process for the student. Patient teaching has been a stimulus for the broader preparation considered essential for the nurse educator in the academic system.

Research Process. The research process provides a method for continual updating of clinical knowledge essential as the scientific base of nursing practice. All types of previous collegiate educational programs in some way prepare the nurse educator for an active role in the research process. Simple problem statements, critiques of articles, investigative activities, statistics, and hands-on computer skills and analysis are the educational preparation for the nursing faculty position. The renewal of knowledge through research is also a criterion of a professional. Quantitative, qualitative, and field research may characterize the nursing research later pursued by nurse educators.

The individual who chooses a professional career as a nurse educator should strive to achieve mastery of these four processes. As basic preliminary skills, these processes are needed for the successful career approach to the larger complex educational system.

The student outcomes of the nurse educator are the teaching, learning, and degrees earned. The outcomes of the process for the nurse educator are of a scholarly nature. If the nurse educator conducts significant research, a role expectation of the body of knowledge essential to improve nursing practice will increase.

Through nursing educational programs at master's and doctoral levels, this knowledge will be tested and further developed by other nurse researchers. The nurse executives and nurse managers of the hospital and community settings seeking higher-level degrees will become more qualified. Further education and more experience are needed by the nursing administrators who direct quality patient care. Priority must be given to the preparation of more educators and leaders to continue the development of the profession (Schlotfeldt, 1982).

Experience

In the ISM, the assessment of the structure also included the experiences that the nurse educator can contribute on entry to the system, especially teaching experience. The experiences of the potential nurse are both personal and professional. These experiences have influenced the nurse educator's maturity, judgment, insight, and decision-making skills. All of the experiences form a foundational bank of knowledge from which to draw on for future career demands as a faculty.

The understanding of self or self-profile is also a part of personal experiences. Likes and dislikes, spare-time activities, and favorite courses and hobbies tell an important story about the nurse educator to an employer. Interests, abilities, and aptitudes can forecast possible work habits. If, during the interview, the candidate can positively address any special talent or skill or reveal flexibility in a situation, the dean may classify the applicant in the group to reinterview.

Age should not be a concern in the search for career entry as a nurse educator; however, appearances that are either too young or too old can affect the choice. The focus for any response to an age-related objection could be a demonstration of the required skill, personality, or energy level sought for the position being filled. The potential new employee who appears eager and ambitious will project a positiveness and willingness to begin a career as a nurse educator. Dressing to project an image is suggested.

Goals

Personal goals are a part of the nurse educator's structure. Personal and professional goal-setting that is planned together is compatible and will enhance the total personality. Matching goals with a realistic self-assessment assists one to identify strengths, weaknesses, preferences, and limitations (Smith, 1982). If independent or highly structured activities are more desirable, the nurse educator can appraise whether this career is realistically the one to select. If certain hours or days are best for coordinating with other family life tasks, knowledge of these are key assessment factors. But many of life's needs for security, social interaction, esteem, autonomy, and self-actualization can be met through a career as a nurse educator.

Goals of a professional nature, which are sought by the individual entering the career field of a nurse educator should help students to meet the objectives and achieve the outcomes of instruction and learning. The personal goals that can be attained are the enrichment of professional life and the rewards of the academic system. Although difficult to measure, citizenship, increased political participation, and development as a community leader have also become goals fulfilled by nurse educators (McPherson, 1983, pp. 240–249).

Values

An initial task in selecting a career is learning about values. Values clarification has been a valuable technique in planning, but is especially important in career planning. Values have influenced the selection of nursing as a professional career and in addition have had even greater influence on the decision for a career as a nurse educator. Some of the values that have influenced career nurse educators were generated from the personal system and individual-needs analysis.

Success in a career as a nurse educator is more likely if there is congruence between both personal and professional values. A need exists for continual assessment of values and their relationship to the professional role. Satisfaction will be influenced by the compatibility between the value system of the nurse and that of the employing institution (Steele & Harmon, 1983).

ASSESSMENT OF THE MARKETPLACE

Following an assessment of individual entry status, the next step of career entry is the assessment of the marketplace. For the nurse educator proposing to seek a position in the college system, it is necessary to learn about the availability and the number of positions, descriptions of the positions, where positions are located, and when the positions are available.

Current resources are available that describe the occupational outlook and predict the feasibility for employment in the field of nursing education. The number of people choosing nursing as an occupation is expected to rise faster than the average for all occupations through the 1990s. The influx is in response to the health care needs for a predicted population of 260 million in 1995 (United States Department of Labor, 1984, 132). This may mean more future positions for nurse faculty.

The new alternatives to health care delivery demand educated nurses. Continual updating of knowledge and skills for the constantly changing client care group is required. A documented need exists for additional nurse educators to also maintain the knowledge and skills base to support nursing leaders in service and practice area (McKibbin, 1983, p. 16).

There was an acute shortage and there continues to be a demand for nurse educators in most settings (Kelly, 1981, p. 292). The outlook is excellent for obtaining positions as doctorally prepared faculty as well as for nurse managers, administrators, and nurses who have degrees in advanced clinical research, community health nursing, or home health care.

A study by a labor economist found professional nursing to be the fifth most desirable occupation of the group studied. When the jobs were ranked according to employment levels, employment growth rates, earning levels, and average unemployment rates, nursing was downgraded only in the area of salaries. The beginning salary ranges were $21,500 to $28,000 for nurse educators, depending on education and experience. If it were not for salary, professional nursing could have been ranked as the most attractive occupation, exceeding engineering, medicine, law, and systems analysis (Walsh, 1982).

With professional nursing by far the highest-ranked traditional women's occupation, women make up 50 percent of the workforce now, and it is estimated for 131 million in 1990. Western and southern areas of the country have been depicted as higher growth sections for future population movement. The increasing aged population group and the growing group of children under 13 years offer other clues to market strategies for nurse educators seeking future career entry (United States Department of Labor, 1984).

The Women's Bureau of the United States Department of Labor has published a guide about federal laws protecting women's rights during job search, employment, and retirement. The section on "Getting the Job" describes legislation that protects and outlines the equal-opportunity complaint process (United States Department of Labor, 1985). State departments of labor, in addition to county and city departments, are also resources for job information and occupational data.

STRATEGIES FOR JOB SEARCH

Since only a short period of time would be required, the obvious first place to look for a new future position is the current location. There are several advantages to securing a promotional or lateral change while remaining with the present institution. Previous knowledge of the system and personnel practices in the current agency will facilitate faster orientation and productivity. Job-searching expenses, telephone calls, resume preparation, and travel time spent in looking elsewhere are decreased. Loss of sick time, vacation time, and other benefits can be prevented.

The disadvantages are familiarity with existing institution, less bargaining power for salary increases, and the difficulties former peers and subordinates may have in accepting the new role.

The job-search strategy of "looking at home" may involve creating a position and marketing the idea to the present employer. The assertiveness in the nurse educator who can negotiate this position will certainly be recognized by administration. To overlook the possibility of continued teaching in the present setting would be unfortunate, even though the present employer may not usually be considered.

Job search is made easy when the nurse educator knows in advance if, where, when, what, and why the new position is offered. A successful job search is more likely if one displays initiative, persistence, seeks referrals from friends, and considers a wider geographical area (Buffie, 1983).

A national study of higher education administrators from over 3000 colleges was conducted. The major reasons found for searching for new positions in academia were the responsibilities of the position, being ready for a change, and the mission or philosophy of the institution. Geographical location, congeniality of colleagues, competency of colleagues, and increased status or prestige were also reasons given for a job search (Moore, 1984).

Study of job search and mobility among nurse educators in the college system determined that the decision to leave the previous job related to a desire for geographical mobility or career advancement and tended not to be motivated by dissatisfaction. Those planning to leave a position rated salary, location of school, and leadership style of the administrator as the most important determinants of the decision to leave (Marriner & Craigie, 1977; Lenz, 1983).

One strategy for job search is to canvass the outstanding universities or medical centers inquiring about the availability of a position as a nurse educator. The more desirable positions at a prestigious college may not be advertised, except by word of mouth, a common communication method. Friends and acquaintances can supply positive recruitment leads.

Prestige is associated with various factors including, but not limited to, the number of faculty, the award of grants, earning accreditation status, research, publications, number of master's and doctoral degrees awarded, amount of federal financial support, size of the endowment, and number of library books. These factors will serve the candidate as content for questions in the interview and provide guidelines for weighing the decision to apply.

Accomplishing the objectives of the mission are included among the critical characteristics of the accredited institution. Meeting student goals or client goals are the barometers of success. Institutional achievement in meeting goals should be reviewed and evaluated by the nurse educator seeking a position in the particular institution (Harris, 1979).

Classified advertising and search agencies have been effectively used for approximately 18 percent of all professional types of positions (Gerberg, 1981). Specialized newspapers known for classified advertisements on positions for nurse educators have included *The American Nurse, The Nation's Health,* and the *Chronicle of Higher Education.* Major city newspapers such as the *Boston Globe,* the *New*

York Times, the *Chicago Tribune,* the *Washington Post,* and the *Los Angeles Times* have a regular coverage of advertisements for nurses at all levels. Local city newspapers are also a source for advertisements, but actually publish only a few for nurse educators.

One of the best sources for employment are the classified advertisements in the professional nursing journals. For nurse educators in the college setting, the best journals to consult are *Nursing Outlook, Journal of Nursing and Health Care, Nursing Research, Nurse Educator,* and *Journal of Nursing Education and Image.* The *American Journal of Nursing, Journal of Nursing Administration, Nursing Management,* and the *American Journal of Public Health* may be reviewed for teaching positions in the college or university settings.

A study of job opportunities for master's-prepared nurses revealed that a total of 6661 advertised positions in nursing were found in 26 national journals over a 3-year period of time between 1978 and 1980. Approximately 50 percent of the positions advertised were for nurses with a master's preparation to enter the educational setting in a school of nursing, while 5.2 percent were for staff development education in the hospital or community.

Although the study was designed to examine the job market for master's-prepared nurses, positions were included, which stated preferences or requirements for doctoral preparation. The number of these positions desiring a doctorate increased from 33 to 50 percent during the period (Balint, 1983).

Circulars and bulletins from institutions provide good information, but are more difficult to obtain unless they can be obtained through a personal network. Some personnel offices will provide a telephone tape service with listings and answer requests for information. Information letters are interchanged between nursing administrators and are posted on faculty and staff bulletin boards. These information letters are often announcements of positions to be offered, and this advance notice is distributed throughout the network of the nursing faculty to all concerned. Again, the friends in various colleges can be aware of this channel of communication to alert any future prospects.

Telephone canvassing, either through the general telephone or college and hospital directories, can be effective. A list can be generated, but this is time consuming and requires preparation. Offering to come in for an interview and requesting that an application be forwarded through the mail are the questions to ask. When any telephone contact is made, care must be taken to obtain the name of the person with whom the conversation transpired for future reference. If an appointment for an interview can be arranged as a result of telephone canvassing, forward a resume in advance with the completed application.

A less used strategy but an effective one for nurse educators is the placement service or employment service. For example, executive search services have assisted nurse educators with job placement. Fees for services may be assessed, and the service is more employer focused, but the advantages are having a wider access to more job openings and the time-saving feature. Civil service recruitment offices do not charge for available listings, but service would probably be more time consuming.

Personal contacts have historically been a rich source of employment referral. This strategy of job search implies the ability to maintain ongoing personal contact with a professional network. A network should be established by the nurse educator throughout the career (Kelly, 1980). Every educational setting or agency where the nurse educator was assigned becomes a pool of potential contacts and for possible references. Personal contacts among faculty and in nursing education should be encouraged.

A network strategy can provide information about positions that are currently available, are about to become available, or are being newly created. Professional contacts will also be able to serve as references in many instances, and because of this potential, need to be nurtured with care. Nursing professionals have been more successful in utilizing networking in the past few years.

Employee referrals are particularly helpful in recruiting, because satisfied employees who are already in the system are very convincing personnel. The inside information and communication channels are most sophisticated mechanisms for advanced scrutiny of a pending position. Internal referrals save valuable time and can expedite the recruitment process.

Attendance at professional and association meetings and presenting papers allow for recruiting and networking of contacts between nurse educators and the nursing administrators attending the meeting. Bulletin boards for messages have served as mini-recruiting centers at the major national nursing conventions. Meetings of other professional disciplines also have served nursing educators as recruiting sources. Local and regional nurses' meetings also provide opportunities for nurse educators to search for openings.

Since 1964, the Council of Baccalaureate and Higher Degree programs of the National League for Nursing has published a continuing source of listings of accredited baccalaureate, master's, and doctoral programs in nursing. These listings are conveniently grouped by state and type of program. While they have provided a convenient method for acquiring career information, they are useful to nurse educators for correspondence because the name, title, and address of the nursing administrators for each program are included (NLN, 1982b; NLN, 1983; NLN, 1985a).

Other NLN publications have been contributed regarding student markets, career choice, faculty role, and collaboration. A group of selected statistical publications have been provided on employment mobility and supply and demand. Anastas (1984) has written a helpful book on a career in nursing.

MARKETING STRATEGIES

If the nurse educator can think of himself or herself as a product to market, three basic market principles can be applied and the strategies of marketing more easily understood. In the self-assessment of individual structure, the nurse educator has identified goals, values, needs, strengths, and weaknesses. Principles of marketing include (Hanger, 1984, p. 19):

- Product knowledge or knowledge of the product
- Knowing the job market to target
- Packaging of the product

Strategies for marketing nurse educators through packaging would include the completion of an application, offering of references and transcripts, preparation of the cover letter, curriculum vitae or resume, interview techniques, and dress.

From the initial telephone conversation to the request for an application to the final interview stages, the employer attempts to seek certain information about the applicant in order to make a decision to hire. If the applicant knows exactly which characteristics are sought in potential candidates, career entry for nurse educators can be better facilitated. The employer will be assessing the structure of the individual nurse educator as in the ISM. Other characteristics in addition to education and experience are applicable to the position for a nurse educator.

Mastery of the subject matter to be taught will be judged. The candidate's choice of career, innate capabilities, potential, initiative, leadership, and professional bearing will be determined throughout the search process. Basic abilities to communicate and work with others are reviewed, and currently assertiveness may be appraised (Nowak & Grindel, 1984). All of the structural qualities of the nurse educator will contribute positively or negatively to the final decision to hire.

Certain attributes or personal qualities and other data should not be communicated or evaluated during the job search process. These data should not be offered by the applicant or questioned by the interviewer. Information such as age, date of birth, religion, gender, marital status, existence of children, credit status, race, color, national origin, or handicap is in this category. A photograph of the applicant is not an appropriate request (Parker, 1984). Other information may be volunteered, for example: hobbies, interests, language skills, and other special skills, if a part of the duties of the position. The answers to these questions should be offered during the interview, when they can be used to an advantage by an application.

References

Both professional and personal references should be offered. A good way to address the process of obtaining professional references is through the services of a placement center. Usually the college where the current degree was earned will offer a reference service without charge. Several professional references, probably between three to five, can be kept on file and released on request to prospective employers.

There are several advantages of this procedure: avoidance of repetitive writing of numerous references by the same group of persons and elimination of retyping and reduction in the mailing time. The persons who are writing the references will appreciate this method; however, references should be updated periodically or every three years. It is suggested that a list of references intended for the application be prepared in advance to give to the interviewer, on request. The list should include the full name and title of the person, complete address, and telephone number.

The written references should differentiate the nurse educator as an outstanding candidate from an average one. Most written references address character, scholarship, responsibility, and competence (Cuthbert, 1977). All recommendations should be written by people who know the characteristics and the teaching ability of the candidate. References should be written by those who write well and will take the time to prepare a significant statement on behalf of the candidate. If a statement is signed to waive the right to read what has been written, some employers believe the reference has more credibility (Buffie, 1983, p. 142).

Personal references numbering at least three should be written by persons who will attest to the maturity level, responsibility, and trustworthiness of the nurse educator. Former supervisors, neighbors, instructors, or colleagues are suitable types of persons for personal references. The employment address, not the home address, should always be used for the personal reference unless the person is unemployed or retired.

Whenever possible, the nurse educator should invite persons to write recommendations who can give excellent ones, both in writing and, if requested, by telephone. What people hesitate to include in written references may often be shared on request over the telephone or in person. Candidates should realize many references are obtained in this manner.

Some of the questions answered by the person over the telephone that do not appear in writing on the reference would include many of the following questions: How did the applicant get along with others or with supervisors? Did the applicant have any negative personal habits? Poor attendance? Criminal record? What was the reason for leaving? What were the applicant's strengths and weaknesses? Was the applicant passed over for promotion? Would re-employment be considered (Fortunato & Waddell, 1981, p. 127)? Judicious and confidential telephone calls made to the writers of references will expedite the search process (Nishio, 1977, p. 717).

Transcripts

Transcripts are the acceptable documentation of the educational degrees or certificates. It is usually required that the official transcripts be confidentially sent directly to the employer from the registrar of the institution. Unfortunately, this is a time-consuming process; however, it is necessary. Because of the time involved, transcripts should be requested approximately 8 weeks before the due date. It is suggested that a small fee in the form of a check be sent with the request to better expedite the process. If one does not know the fee, one can ask to be billed. Occasionally, an employer will inquire about the possibility of viewing an unofficial copy of the transcript with the understanding the official one will be forthcoming. In this case, the nurse educator may share a personal copy for review at the interview.

Preparation of the Cover Letter

A cover letter must accompany the curriculum vitae or resume of the nurse educator who is seeking employment. The purpose of the cover letter is to formally introduce the nurse educator as an applicant and to express an interest in a specific position.

The cover letter should be short, approximately 150 words, and typed perfectly on good-quality bond paper. It should "cover" or precede the formal information contained on the resume, which is enclosed with it.

The cover letter should be addressed to a specific person whose name is correctly spelled and whose title is accurate and not abbreviated. If this information is not made available on the advertisement, an effort must be made to obtain this information over the telephone. To err in this aspect will have a negative effect on the candidate. To address the letter "To whom it may concern" or to address the position, i.e. "Dear Dean" or "Dear Director of Nurses," should be avoided.

Two sample cover letters have been provided (Figs. 6–1 and 6–2). The first cover letter (Fig. 6–1) is in response to an advertised position and should attract the attention of the prospective employer. It should be convincing enough to grant the candidate's request for an interview. The second sample (Fig. 6–2) is used when there is no specific opening but the nurse educator wishes to contact an employer about the possibility of an opening in a specific type of position.

Both the solicited and the unsolicited cover letter are to be prepared on plain

---

1010 Parsimmon Road
Brice, IN 26132
November 10, 1986

Dr. Laverne Fields
Dean, School of Nursing
The State University of the South
Austin, TX 66666

Dear Dr. Fields,

With an interest in a faculty position in the school of nursing, I am writing in reference to the position advertised in the *Nursing Outlook* for an Assistant Professor in Medical Surgical nursing.

During the past three years I have been an Instructor in staff education at Brice Memorial Medical Center. My educational background has also prepared me for this position. In 1986, I earned a Master's of Science in nursing with role preparation for teaching.

I have enclosed my curriculum vitae for your review. I would enjoy meeting with you and discussing the teaching position. I will call for an appointment next week. References will be provided on request.

Sincerely yours,

Joan Bennett, M.S., R.N.

Figure 6–1. Sample cover letter 1.

Monica Johnson, M.S.N., R.N.
2414 South Main St.
Northford, Mo. 03921
(400) 371-5620

April 10, 1986

Dr. Bernice Flaven, Ph.D., R.N.
Dean, School of Nursing
Southwest University
100 University Parkway
Phoenix, Arizona 17317

Dear Dr. Flaven,

I am inquiring about the possibility of a position as an Assistant Professor in the School of Nursing at Southwest University.

I earned my Master of Science in nursing three years ago and have been teaching in a baccalaureate program in nursing, which has prepared me for this type of position. My resume is attached.

I am available for an interview, and I will call you next week to arrange an appointment if this is convenient for you. Thank you for your kind attention. I am looking forward to meeting you.

Sincerely,

Monica Johnson, M.S.N., R.N.

Figure 6–2. Sample cover letter 2.

paper or paper with a personal letterhead. If available, the nurse educator may use personalized business stationery or personal stationery and enclose a calling card.

The writing style of the cover letter should be direct, powerful, and free of grammar, spelling, or punctuation errors. Paragraph one should contain statements of purpose and interest. The second paragraph should highlight the enclosed resume and focus on what the employer can expect from the candidate in the position. The use of a formal but friendly tone, which is sincere but not overenthusiastic is suggested (Kelly, 1981, p. 634). The content should be a positive expression of past accomplishments. However, pointing out the future value of the candidate is recommended.

The final paragraph should request the interview appointment and state a date and time when a follow-up telephone inquiry will be made regarding a specific appointment. The accepted complimentary close for the cover letter is either "Sincerely yours" or "Sincerely," as for a business letter. If the nurse educator has professional calling cards available, it is convenient to clip one to the top of the cover letter.

Keeping current records of the job-search activity and progress will be essential. When multiple positions are being considered and approached simultaneously, positions, contact persons, and dates are easily confused. A system for filing should be developed, which is simple but efficient. The name of contact person, address, telephone number with dates of contact, application deadline, resume sent date, transcript sent date, references sent date, the appointment date, and other search committee activities should be included. A note regarding the status of the offer (either pending, yes, or not offer), and whether a thank-you note has been sent are valuable entries (Nowak & Grindel, 1984, pp. 109–111).

Curriculum Vitae

A resume or curriculum vitae is the documentation of a career. A well-written resume is essential to a successful job search, and it must effectively describe education, experience, achievements, and expertise. It is a brief, typed, double-spaced summary of qualifications and skills used in applying for positions. A resume is a relatively short biography. In academic settings, a curriculum vitae (CV), which is lengthier and contains different, more detailed information, is the appropriate form of professional biography (Newcomb, 1979).

The usual format of the CV is the reverse chronological order type (Fig. 6–3). The following categories are included:

- Identifying data
    Name with title
    Address with city and zip code
    Telephone numbers at work and at home (with complete area codes and extensions)
- License and registration number
    State
    Expiration date
- Education
    Name, address of postsecondary institutions attended with dates
    Name of degree, date granted, and content area of degree
- Certification, date awarded, content area, and expiration date
- Experience
    Title of position
    Name
    Address of employer and beginning and end date
    Description of duties and responsibilities
- Military assignments
- Honors and awards
- Research and grants
- Professional memberships with committees
    Offices held, place and dates

Marlene Louise Moore 3131 Peachtree Lane Pleasantville, Montana 21221 (171) 826-2131	Instructor American College (171) 827-6543

EDUCATION

R.N. license 731234567 (optional) Colorado, exp. January 1987	Certification: Medical-Surgical Nursing May 1986, exp. May 1989
B.S. Nursing September 1976 to May 1980	Southwest University 1000 Campus Drive Rivertown, Nebraska 17818
M.S. Nursing May 1982 to June 1984	University for the Americas 5 University Place Denver, Colorado 37373

EXPERIENCE

Staff nurse on 27-bed surgical unit, relief charge week-ends May 1980 to May 1982	Midtown Hospital 117 N. Main Street Rivertown, Nebraska 17818
Instructor in medical-surgical nursing: nursing diagnosis course July 1984 to June 1986	American College 481 Jefferson Way Centerville, Montana 71819

AWARDS
Graduated Cum Laude, Southwest University
May 1980

PROFESSIONAL MEMBERSHIPS

American Nurses' Association Sigma Theta Tau	Member since May 1980 June 1984

RESEARCH
Moore, M.L. (1986). An Analysis of Pain Management in Postoperative Orthopedic Surgery Patients. Operating Room Nurses, 7(2), 17–21.

CONTINUING EDUCATION

Trauma Course 2 CEUs June 1985	Division of Nursing State College Downey, Idaho 17812
CPR Certification April 1986	American Heart Association Centerville, Montana 71819

Figure 6–3. Sample curriculum vitae.

- Papers and presentations
- Consultation
- Publications (in the format of the American Psychological Association)
- Continuing education
    List credits or CEUs
    Dates
    Places
- References

For the less experienced nurse, not all of these categories will be used. A summary page of significant contributions has been an option when the CV is particularly lengthy or to briefly highlight the important items. A treatment of a professional goal is also optional.

Interview

A nurse educator who communicates skillfully during the interview adds an important dimension to the list of qualifications. The theory of communication has been stressed in nursing and nursing education. Communication is one of the four processes of the nurse educator in the ISM. Nurse educators who effectively utilize these skills during the job search have increased the opportunities for surpassing the competition and obtaining the position. Good listening skills are a part of communication, and listening will project an honest concern and strong interest in the position.

The interview is an opportunity for the candidate and the potential employer to gather information. Both asking questions and answering questions accurately will further enhance the interaction between the interviewed and the interviewer. Some examples of information gathering by the applicant would include the inquiries about the future and the security of the position and the salary, benefits, and hours (Swansburg & Swansburg, 1984, p. 196).

Prior to the interview, it would be wise to obtain background information through research on the community. Read in advance the local newspaper and the literature about the institution, the college catalog, course schedule, and the hospital or community information brochures about services. If it is possible to drive to the place of the interview as a practice activity, locating both the building and parking arrangements ahead of time should reduce the stress on the day of the interview.

Preparation for the interview should include modeling the total outfit to be worn in front of the mirror. Wear exactly what will be worn during the interview, avoiding any anxiety about new clothes or accessories. Select conservative styles, and choose the colors suited for complexion and hair. A photograph might be interesting.

Role-playing with a colleague prior to the interview can be helpful. Use of videotaping with playback, which can be erased later, is very convincing. Have well-researched and rehearsed comments on professional goals, interests, and strengths prepared. The nurse educator should recall a philosophy of nursing education and what encompasses good teaching. Offering information about continuing education achievements or professional volunteer work would be strongly positive.

Nurse educators should ask questions about salary, schedules, fringe benefits, and other job conditions (i.e., audiovisual equipment, current texts for nursing courses, film rental, and library holdings). Other inquiries can be made relevant to office space, committees, student enrollment, and starting date. However, the most appropriate questions should be philosophy-centered rather than benefit-centered. The responses to the open-ended questions asked by the interviewer should sound spontaneous and natural (Talento, 1983). For the interviewer, index cards may be comfortable to use, with important dates and pertinent information for quick reference.

Nonverbal communication is important as well. The handshake may be given on arrival and when leaving. A calling card may be presented. Nervous mannerisms should be avoided, but eye contact should be maintained as much as can be tolerated. Body movements (i.e., wiggling, leg pumping, flushed or pale facial appearance, diaphoresis, or clenched fists), may demonstrate anxiety to others. A flat effect would also be observed and could be evaluated negatively in an interview.

Body positions reveal attitudes and give impressions. Open positions with hands and feet relaxed show receptivity. Hands and feet close to the body or closing off the body suggest tension and defensiveness. Duplication of the other's position, however, can signify agreement (Davis, 1984).

Nonverbal behavior can have significant impact on perceived effectiveness of the nurse educator applicant and could affect hiring decisions. High-level direct gaze, frequent smiling, and hand gestures were characteristics found in successful engineering applicants (Forbes, 1980). In addition, gestures and head nods by applicants produced favorable hiring decisions (Patterson, 1983). A degree of personal power can be communicated nonverbally through demonstrating self-confidence, having a well-dressed appearance, and behaving formally (Lamar, 1985).

To market oneself as a nurse educator, remember the ABCs of the first impression:

- Appearance
- Behavior
- Communication

Although basic characteristics, all are vital in the job selection of a candidate. Listen carefully and answer questions concisely. Refrain from smoking and talking incessantly. Refuse offers for beverages unless you can efficiently manipulate containers, note cards, and personal belongings. Brief notetaking is appropriate if you are invited to tour the institution. Do so, as it will probably serve as an opportunity to learn more about the setting. The interview will probably consume 40 to 45 minutes. Recall the principles of product marketing; only a brief time exists to sell the product: the nurse educator candidate.

Currently, interviews for positions in college settings are conducted by more than one person or by a search committee. The search committee is composed of between three to five members, and the search process may be extended to two days (Nowak & Grindel, 1984). "Searchwiseness" is an asset to the nurse educator during the group interview process. The searchwise candidate appears well poised, is dressed in a suit or tailored dress, and has a predetermined battery of the "right" questions and answers (Heller, 1982). The searchwise candidates do their homework, review the mission of the college and the curriculum materials, and can articulate how they can make a contribution to the nursing program. They are able to weave their research abilities and grantsmanship into the dialogue. They have the ability to anticipate the situational-type questions and to respond appropriately. The candidate may be asked to problem solve a set of situations usually found in the student–faculty or teaching–learning relationships. For example: how to motivate students, or how to design curriculum or test questions.

The recruitment process for the higher ranks of associate or full professor may involve the presentation of research, or a seminar may be requested as part of the formal agenda. Meetings with students, faculty, or faculty from other disciplines and clinical nursing personnel are usually reserved for candidates who will have administrative responsibilities (Hawken, 1979).

When the search committee process is used, the questions regarding salary, fringe benefits, community service, and tenure eligibility may be addressed in committee but are the responsibility of the dean (Poteet, 1983). After review of the candidate, the search committee makes a recommendation, and the final decision to hire rests with the dean (Bayne, 1982). Once the interview has taken place, the nurse educator should send a formal thank-you note to the administrator.

In the past, factors that have influenced faculty to select a position and to remain in it have included: opportunity to utilize one's own knowledge and skills in an area of choice, nature of teaching load and assignment, availability of clinical facilities for student learning experiences, and curriculum of programs and opportunities for continued education through formal courses (Seyfried, 1977). The opportunity to conduct research is a deciding factor (NLN, 1985b).

If the position is offered, a letter offering the position with a contract for signature will be sent stating the parameters of the position, title, salary, and starting date. The contract should be signed and returned promptly. Since recruitment, selection, and retention demand much time, nurse educators who understand the expectations at the start will be better able to know when and where and how they will be met.

Any selection of competent nurse educators for teaching positions in the college system is a crucial and time-consuming process. The compatibility between the institution and the nurse educator applicant hopefully will result in the desired position being filled. Entry into the career as a nurse educator requires a thorough understanding of the role in order to accomplish the responsibilities of the position.

REFERENCES

Anastas, L. (1984). *Your career in nursing.* New York: National League for Nursing.
Andreoli, K., & Musser, L. (1985). Trends that may affect nursing's future. *Nursing and Health Care, 6*(1), 47–51.
Balint, J. (1983). Job opportunities for master's prepared nurses. *Nursing Outlook, 31,* 109–114.
Bayne, M. (1982). The search committee process. *Nursing Outlook, 30,* 178–181.
Bolles, N. (1980). *What color is your parachute: A practical manual for job-hunters and career changers* (p. 100). Berkeley, Calif.: Ten Speed Press.
Brademas, J. (Ed.). (1983). *Signs of trouble and erosion: A report on graduate education in America* (pp. 27, 65, 78). New York University: National Commission on Student Financial Assistance.
Brown, B., & Chinn, P. (1982). *Nursing education: Practical methods and models* (p. 66). Rockville, Md.: Aspen.
Buffie, E. (1983). Strategies for a successful job search. *Educational Horizons, 61,* 140–143.

Butterfield, S. (1985). Professional nursing education: What is its purpose. *Journal of Continuing Education, 24*(3), 99–102.

Conway, M., & Andruskiw, O. (1983). *Administrative theory and practice: Issues in higher education* (p. 371). E. Norwalk, Conn.: Appleton-Century-Crofts.

Cuthbert, B. (1977). Please list three names. *The American Journal of Nursing, 77,* 1596–1599.

Davis, A. (1984). Body talk. *The American Journal of Nursing, 84,* 932–933.

Ehrat, K. (1981). Educational/career mobility: Antecedent of change. *Nursing and Health Care, 11,* 487–527.

Flanagan, M. (1981). *Summary of the public hearings* (pp. 15, 29–30). National Commission on Nursing. Chicago: The Hospital Research and Educational Trust.

Forbes, R. (1980). Nonverbal behavior and outcome of selection interview. *Journal of Occupational Psychology, 53,* 65–72.

Fortunato, R., & Waddell, D. (1981). *Personnel administration in higher education* (p. 127). San Francisco: Jossey-Bass Publishers.

Gerberg, R. (1981). *The professional job changing system* (pp. 7, 16, 27). Parsippany, N.J.: Performance Dynamics.

Hanger, T. (1984). How to market yourself. In *The AJN Guide: A Review of Nursing Career Opportunities in 1984* (pp. 19–23). New York: American Journal of Nursing Company.

Harris, J. (1979). How do you know a good college when you stumble over one? *Current Issues in Higher Education, 5,* 35–38.

Hawken, P. (1979). Faculty recruitment or after the advertisement. *Nursing Outlook, 27,* 420–422.

Heller, B. (1982). The search interview. *Nursing Outlook, 30,* 182–185.

Kelly, L. (1980). Contacts. *Nursing Outlook, 28,* 396.

Kelly, L. (1981). *Dimensions of professional nursing* (4th ed.) (pp. 292, 626–641). New York: Macmillan.

Kelly, L. (1985). Strategic planning for the 1990s. *Nursing Outlook, 33*(8).

Keough, G. (1977). Faculty development. *Current Issues in Higher Education, 2,* 29–32.

Lamar, E. (1985). Communicating personal power through nonverbal behavior. *Journal of Nursing Administration,* 41–44.

Lenz, E. (1983). Patterns of job search and mobility among nurse educators. *Journal of Nursing Education, 22,* 267–273.

Marriner, A., & Craigie, D. (1977). Job satisfaction and mobility of nursing educators in baccalaureate and higher degree programs in the west. *Nursing Research, 26,* 349–360.

McKibbin, R. (1983). *Economic and employment issues in nursing education* (p. 16). Kansas City: American Nurses' Association.

McPherson, M. (1983). Value conflicts in American higher education: A survey. *The Journal of Higher Education, 54,* 243–278.

Moore, K. (1984). *Leaders in transition: A national study of higher education administrators.* University Park, Pa.: American Council on Education and Pennsylvania State University.

National League for Nursing. (1981). *Position statement on preparation for practice in nursing.* New York: National League for Nursing.

National League for Nursing. (1982a). *Position statement of educational mobility.* New York: National League for Nursing.

National League for Nursing (1982b). *Baccalaureate education in nursing: Key to a professional career in nursing, 1982–83* (Pub. No. 15-1311). New York: NLN Council on Baccalaureate and Higher Degree Programs.

National League for Nursing. (1983). *Master's education in nursing: Route to opportunities in contemporary nursing, 1983–84* (Pub. No. 15-1312). New York: NLN Council on Baccalaureate and Higher Degree Programs.

National League for Nursing. (1985a). *Doctoral programs in nursing* (Pub. No. 15-1448). New York: National League for Nursing.

National League for Nursing. (1985b). *NLN continuing education programs.* New York: National League for Nursing.

Newcomb, J. (1979). The curriculum vitae: What it is and what it is not. *Nursing Outlook, 27,* 580–583.

Nishio, K. (1977). The right and the qualified. *Nursing Outlook, 25,* 713–717.

Nowak, J., & Grindel, C. (1984). *Career planning in nursing.* Philadelphia: Lippincott.

Parker, M. (1984). How to write your resume. In *The AJN Guide: A Review of Nursing Career Opportunities in 1984.* New York: American Journal of Nursing Company.

Patterson, M. (1983). *Nonverbal behavior: A functional perspective.* New York: Springer Verlag.

Poteet, G. (1983). Planning successful academic interviews. *Nurse Educator, 8*(2), 11–14.

Schlotfeldt, R. (1982). The significance of academic preparation (editorial). *Nursing Papers, 14*(4), 2–9.

Schwirian, P. (1981). Toward an explanatory model of nursing performance. *Nursing Research, 30,* 247–253.

Seyfried, S. (1977). Factors influencing faculty choice of position. *Nursing Outlook, 25,* 592–696.

Shane, D. (1983). *Returning to school: A guide for nurses.* Englewood Cliffs, N.J.: Prentice-Hall.

Smith, M. (1982). Career development in nursing: An individual and professional responsibility. *Nursing Outlook, 30,* 128–131.

Steele, S., & Harmon, V. (1983). Values clarification in nursing (2nd ed.) (pp. 7–9, 84). E. Norwalk, Conn.: Appleton-Century-Crofts.

Swansburg, R., & Swansburg, P. (1984). *Strategic career planning and development for nurses.* Rockville, Md.: Aspen.

Talento, B. (1983). Improving interviewing techniques. *Nursing Outlook, 31,* 234–235.

United States Department of Labor. (1984). *Occupational outlook handbook, 1984–85* (p. 132). Washington, D.C.: Bureau of Labor Statistics.

United States Department of Labor. (1985). *A working woman's guide to her job rights.* Washington, D.C.: Women's Bureau.

Walsh, P. (1982). Comparing occupations: Four measures. *Occupational Outlook Quarterly* (Fall), 27–30.

White, D. (1983, July). HRSA predicts health professions balance by 2000. *Washington Actions on Health.*

7

Rewards and Risks

Patricia D. Scearse, D.N.Sc., R.N.

NURSING EDUCATION SYSTEMS

The 2979 nursing programs in the United States provide over 60,000 positions for nursing faculty throughout the country (American Nurses Association, 1985, p. 152; Rosenfeld, 1987, p. 286). Nurses choose to seek and accept teaching positions for many different reasons. Some of the reasons for seeking teaching appointments are more likely to result in jobs and professional satisfaction than others.

Most nurse educators understand and probably value education as a tool for social system change. Nurses who come to believe that change will not occur in service agencies sometimes seek positions in educational institutions as a possible solution. Others may value research activities and outcomes, and believe that academic life will support and sustain those interests. Many professional nurses have held teaching positions as lifelong goals and believe their talents are best used in transmitting knowledge and skills to the next cohort of professionals. A few may perceive a position in higher education as a part-time position demanding nine months' service instead of twelve, and further view an educational position as one, which offers flexible hours and routines. and which will enable them to better fulfill other important roles in their lives. These roles may include graduate student, parent, spouse, community volunteer worker, or a combination of any of those listed.

American systems of higher education are unique and complex, and thus hold sets of purposes, functions, goals, and values that are for the most part unrelated to the individual goals of faculty members. It is very important that first-time faculty aspirants carefully examine the position, the system, and their motivation. The rewards to be derived or that may be bestowed by any educational system are not as varied or diverse as the needs and desires of faculty members employed by the system.

COLLEGE NURSING PROGRAMS

Surrounding nursing educators today is a seething turmoil of disagreement concerning the products of the various nursing educational programs and how they should be titled, licensed, and used in the health care arena. The importance of this turmoil to seekers of first-time faculty positions cannot be understated. There is not a true educational ladder operating for students. Faculty who seek first teaching positions in educational settings other than colleges and universities may find in future years that the previous years of teaching may not serve as a positive factor in resumes. Indeed, the years may act as a negative factor in the credential review. For that reason, nurses seeking positions as faculty in nursing schools should familiarize themselves with the various types and forms of nursing programs existing today and the existing conflicts among them.

The baccalaureate degree program in nursing prepares the student to become an entry-level professional nurse. Housed in colleges and universities, most baccalaureate-degree programs are four years in length, and the nursing component is taught in the last two or three years. These programs are often referred to as *upper division nursing programs*. Baccalaureate programs may be located in institutions that also offer master's programs or master's and doctoral programs.

Faculty applicants may expect significant differences in employment expectations and institutional policies between institutions that have both graduate and undergraduate nursing programs and those, which offer only a baccalaureate program.

In recent years, institutions have developed *registered nurse completion programs*. These offer to registered nurses who are graduates of diploma or associate-degree programs a specifically designed upper-division curriculum that is generally completed in 12 to 15 months, after all lower-division prerequisites have been completed. These students often obtain credit in many courses by examination.

An entry-level nursing education program, which offers the *Nursing Doctorate* (N.D.) has been implemented at Case Western University in Cleveland, Ohio. This controversial program is being perceived by many as an educational model for entry into professional practice, and several colleges and universities are now considering the establishment of similar degree programs.

The various types of initial nursing programs have a common stated outcome: the preparation of a generalist at the entry level of nursing practice. Although this is true, there is little if any agreement about the appropriateness, merit, or quality of the graduates of these different types of programs. A fierce competition is developing for qualified faculty, and concern is sometimes expressed by administrators in the programs housed in 4-year colleges and universities about philosophical differences in educational approaches to nursing education that may become critical in selection of faculty for the upper-division nursing programs.

All nursing programs whose graduates are allowed to write the licensing examinations for registered nurses (R.N.) must be approved by the state licensing agency designated by state law. National accreditation of a nursing education program, however, is a voluntary action and is only one indicator of quality.

While every program that seeks and receives voluntary accreditation has met certain quality standards, many programs with equally high standards may choose not to seek accreditation for a variety of reasons. For example, the administration of the institution may consider the costs involved to be prohibitive. Choosing to teach in a nonaccredited program, regardless of quality, is a decision that should be considered very carefully if a future in nursing education in a prestige institution is a professional goal. As of 1984, 96 percent (269) of the diploma, 81 percent (352) of the baccalaureate, and 54 percent (421) of the associate-degree programs were nationally accredited by the National League for Nursing (ANA, 1985, p. 118).

REWARD SYSTEMS OF EDUCATIONAL INSTITUTIONS

Rewards available from educational systems are limited in scope, and the decisions negotiated at the time of initial appointment may have far-reaching impact on individual faculty members. The rewards for the nurse educator include rank, salary, promotion, tenure, assignments, and a variety of benefits.

Initial Salary and Rank

Institutions vary considerably in the freedom or latitude the dean of a nursing program has to negotiate an entry-appropriate level and salary. (The term "dean" is used to denote the academic unit head. The actual title may be dean, director, coordinator, or head.) Usually public institutions have fixed salary schedules with steps and levels, and there are designated education levels and experiential credentials appropriate to each of these steps and levels. Although many private institutions also use similar schedules, many do not, and the need of the institution for the individual candidate or the urgency within the system to fill the position may influence the initial offer in such cases. Basically, all deans will look at the same qualifications:

- Education, including graduate preparation in nursing in the clinical or theory area of the position to be filled and preparation in the functional role of teaching. Educational credits past the master's or an earned doctorate in nursing or a closely related field is becoming increasingly important to college and university programs for tenure-track positions.
- Nursing experience in a clinical setting appropriate to the position. Although programs differ in the weight given to this qualification, all nursing education programs desire faculty to be clinically capable. Some programs may demand clinical experience following the completion of the master's degree, believing that advanced clinical preparation and knowledge must be practiced at least in some limited fashion prior to teaching. This is especially true in graduate programs.

- Teaching experience is probably the area of greatest variance in the credit allowed for previous professional experience. Some systems will credit as years of experience *any* teaching position in any school of nursing. Other systems will credit only teaching done in approved or accredited institutions of higher education. Still others will credit only teaching experience, which followed the earned master's or earned doctoral degree. This may be a point of negotiation at the time of employment. The number of credited years of teaching experience may influence both entry salary level and credit towards tenure.

Generally, nursing schools that have well-established graduate and undergraduate programs have less difficulty in attracting faculty applicants. Also, more fixed policies exist. Programs that encounter difficulty in attracting qualified and credentialed faculty may have greater freedom to negotiate the initial appointment.

It is helpful for the faculty candidate to obtain a faculty roster that indicates highest degrees held, academic rank, and date of employment of currently employed faculty. Many college and university catalogues include such information. It is then possible to assess where the credentials of the applicant may fit into the system.

Some public university systems have on file at the university library a listing of all faculty salaries for the current year; other systems have step-and-level salary scales available. State institution salaries are a matter of public record and are made available to those requesting this information. This information may or may not be available at private institutions.

Faculty candidates may also profit by obtaining the Faculty Salary Survey report published annually by the American Association of Colleges of Nursing (1986–1987) located at One Dupont Circle, Suite 530, Washington, D.C. 20036. These data are presented by rank for geographic regions, doctoral and nondoctoral preparation, and for private and public institutions.

Tenure

Defined as an arrangement under which faculty appointments in an institution of higher education are continued until retirement for age or physical disability, subject to dismissal for adequate cause or unavoidable termination on account of financial exigency or change of institutional programs, probably no one issue has more force or impact upon an educational system than tenure. Probably no one concept is more misunderstood. It is important for prospective faculty to seek information about and try to understand:

- The minimum qualifications for tenure
- How tenure is achieved (process)
- How tenure decisions are made
- Where a written document concerning tenure can be located

All too often novice faculty members accept positions "on the tenure track" with little understanding that criteria for achieving a successful final tenure review far exceed mere satisfactory teaching performance. Most frequently abused by the tenure-track system in universities are faculty prepared at the master's level who may be expected to:

- Obtain a doctorate
- Establish a consistent publication record
- Participate in professional organizations and community activities
- Engage in and publish the results of research activities
- Successfully fulfill the faculty role in classroom and clinical settings

All of this must be accomplished in a relatively short period of time, usually not exceeding seven years.

At the time of employment, many new nursing faculty seem to view "any credit toward tenure" as a down payment on the total cost of tenure. In reality, credit toward tenure granted at the time of employment may act as a negative factor in achieving tenure by significantly reducing the time available to conduct and publish the results of research and establish a consistent record of scholarly activities. "The tenure apparatus is . . . not designed for the individual but for the institution. It is an apparatus whose purpose is to enable the institution over the years to define itself, to speak to the wider community as to what it is, what it stands for. . . ." (Morris, 1981, p. 62). The institution so defines itself and speaks through the decisions made about faculty who are and are not tenured. University administration speaks of the tenure decision as a multimillion-dollar decision after calculating that a university faculty member earning tenure at age 35 is assured of a salary for 35 years. Only with this information can any nontenured faculty assess the probability of achieving tenure within a given institution.

Questions about tenure that prospective or new faculty may find worth pursuing include:

- Is there a mechanism by which the tenure clock may be "stopped" after initial employment?
- What previous tenure "credit," if any, will be "given" at the time of employment?
- When will the final tenure review occur?

It is also important for prospective faculty to read the faculty handbook.

The practice of awarding tenure at the time of initial employment has virtually disappeared. In rare cases, it may be granted by a system to a highly desirable candidate who has previously achieved tenure in another institution. In such cases, the offer of tenure can be used as a negotiating point when questions of salary and rank are at an impasse.

Salary Increments and Promotion

In addition, issues of salary increments and promotion in rank are important to faculty job satisfaction and retention. Annual salary increments are determined either under a cost-of-living (COLA) system, a merit system, or, most likely, a combination of both. The administrator will determine the extent to which salaries within a given institution will follow the pre-existing salary steps. The pre-existing "steps" or schedules are generated by length of service, rather than merit.

In a rigorous step-and-level system, the dean may have little decision making. In other systems where there is virtually no outside limit on the percentage increase to any one individual salary, adjustments are made related to the pool of money available. Table 7–1 depicts increases in dollars and in percentages under four different distribution criteria. Under Option A, the institution has mandated a 2.5 COLA increase. The dean has distributed the remaining monies in percentages ranging from 2.5 to 5 percent. No faculty member could receive less than a 2.5 percent increase, and as the dean distributed the merit monies, no faculty member received less than 5 percent.

In Options B, C, and D, however, all monies were made available for "merit" increases. Under Option B, the dean decided that faculty member C was an underachiever and awarded *no* salary increase. The $5000 was distributed heavily to the faculty in lower ranks to "make the positions competitive." A lesser percentage was then available to faculty members D and E, who held senior ranks. Under Option C, the merit money was distributed as a 5-percent "across-the-board" increase. The dean must have believed all faculty members were performing at an equal quality level.

In Option D, $1000 was given to each faculty member, possibly due to a "fairness" criterion. (If everyone is underpaid, all should share equally.) This resulted, however, in percentage increases, which ranged from 3.3 percent for senior faculty to 10 percent for junior faculty (Table 7–1).

The above examples indicate the importance of individual faculty members having access to the *criteria* for merit considerations and an understanding of the basis on which merit decisions are made and by whom they are made.

Basic Fringe Benefits

Benefits do not differ significantly in kind among employers of full-time faculty. Generally, provisions are made for life insurance, Social Security contribution, health insurance, and perhaps hospital insurance, which may or may not include dental coverage. (Some nonprofit organizations have opted out of Social Security and list this as a benefit because employees do not contribute. Careful consideration of the cost–benefit of this is urged for individuals without a disability insurance or retirement system.)

Some systems offer generous retirement contributions, and sometimes the starting date for such contributions is a negotiable item at employment. There may be a waiting period for entry into the benefit plan, which at times can be negotiated. Obviously, if the employer contributes 10 percent of the basic salary to an employee-owned retirement plan, the starting date for entry into the plan can be a significant salary item.

Other benefits sometimes available include liability (malpractice) insurance coverage or premium reimbursement, tuition reimbursement for the faculty member

TABLE 7-1. MERIT INCREASE EXAMPLES UNDER DIFFERENT DISTRIBUTION CRITERIA

	Present Salary $	COLA $	Option A[a] Merit $	Option A[a] %	Total $	Option B[b] Merit $	Option B[b] %	Option C[b] Merit $	Option C[b] %	Option D[b] Merit $	Option D[b] %
Faculty											
A	10,000	250	250	2.5	500	1000	10.0	500	5.0	1000	10.0
B	15,000	375	375	2.5	750	1500	10.0	750	5.0	1000	6.6
C	20,000	500	1000	5.0	1500	—	—	1000	5.0	1000	5.0
D	25,000	625	—	—	625	1300	5.2	1250	5.0	1000	4.0
E	30,000	750	875	2.9	1625	1200	4.0	1500	5.0	1000	3.3
Totals	100,000	2500	2500		5000	5000		5000		5000	

Faculty N=5; Total salary budget = $100,000; Money available for increases = 5% or $5000.
[a]2.5% COLA required.
[b]No COLA required.

TABLE 7-2. BENEFITS CHECKLIST

- Life insurance
- Social Security contributions
- Health or hospital insurance
- Dental coverage
- Disability insurance
- Retirement
- Liability insurance (malpractice)
- Premium reimbursement
- Tuition reimbursements for faculty; for dependents
- University automobiles
- Mileage reimbursement for travel
- Sabbatical leaves
- Reimbursement for attending professional meetings
- Release time for
    Pursuit of advanced degree
    Unfunded research activities
- Services of
    Secretarial support
    Computer center
    Library
- Office space
- Parking

and the spouse (and sometimes dependent children) of the faculty member, university automobiles for use to travel to remote clinical sites, and earned sabbatical leaves. Written statements on all such policies are easily obtained from the university personnel office. It is helpful to have a checklist of these benefits on an index card as a tool for prospective faculty during the interview process (Table 7-2).

Other Benefits

Even if not immediately available to new faculty, policies and eligibility for other benefits should be explored during pre-employment interviews. Such benefits include reimbursement for attending professional meetings, services of work-study or graduate assistants, secretary support services, secretarial services for projects outside the teaching role (research, professional activities, community activities), postage and other mailing costs for research activities, computer support, and space.

Although mentioned last, space may be the key to a productive faculty experience. The difference between private and shared offices and additional space for research or project activities can be critical factors in a faculty member's productivity. Whether or not an institution provides such benefits is a clue to how seriously the institution takes its responsibilities in faculty development and advancement.

One added benefit, which may be available to faculty, is release time for pursuit of an advanced degree or for unfunded research activities. This is a very important benefit for faculty who are seeking employment on a tenure track before they have completed the doctoral degree and prior to obtaining any funds for research activities. A clear understanding between the faculty and the school administrator at the time of employment can prevent a serious misunderstanding from occurring later.

Intrinsic Rewards of an Academic Institution

Not all the rewards gained by employment as a faculty member come in the form of money, space, or physical accoutrements. Although at times severely questioned, a position on a college or university faculty carries with it a status and credibility. Working environments, both physical and collegial, may well be superior to other work environments. Access to cultural and social activities related to the university is a significant but often overlooked benefit. The opportunity to meet with and associate with a host of visiting dignitaries, scholars. and campus visitors affords opportunities unavailable in other settings. Involvement of the family in university-related activities such as sports events, recitals, plays, and lectures is usually free or available at a greatly reduced fee. The university environment is generally a healthy, congenial, exciting place to be.

FACTORS INFLUENCING REWARDS AND RISKS

Contracts

Generally, contracts are issued by all employing institutions to nontenured faculty and should be examined with extreme care prior to signing. Regardless of verbal "understandings" negotiated with the dean, the parameters of the position will be as set forth in the contract. In most instances, the contract will not originate from or be signed by the dean, but rather by the chief academic officer of the institution. The contract should clearly set forth certain items such as:

- Beginning and ending dates
- Salary for time period of contract
- Number of payments to be made
- Administrator of the employing unit
- Benefits and starting date for each benefit
- Nature of contract

The *nature* of the contract is in respect to either term: renewable, probationary, multiyear, part-time, or full-time, the benefits to be awarded, and the starting dates of each benefit. Many times such contracts will refer to a faculty handbook or policy manual. Faculty applicants must make certain such documents have been made available and have been read thoroughly. If an agreement exists regarding moving expenses or other pre-employment benefits, a statement must be contained in the contract document. It should not be assumed that an incorrect statement in a proposed contract is an error that can be corrected after the contract is signed and employment has begun.

Collective Bargaining

Collective bargaining and union membership are increasingly important facets of faculty life in institutions where personnel policies are determined through formal bargaining and group contracting. Under such circumstances, virtually all the information in this chapter, which has preceded this section is irrelevant.

The 1947 Labor Management Relations Act, often referred to as the Taft–Hartley Bill, defined collective bargaining as:

> . . . the performance of the mutual obligation of the employers and representatives of employees to meet at reasonable times and confer in good faith with respect to wages, hours and other terms and conditions of employment . . . and the execution of a written contract incorporating any agreement reached . . . (Baker, 1983, p. 780).

The process and roles of individuals involved in collective bargaining for colleges and universities differ depending on the organization's status as a private or public, large or small institution. However, in all cases collective bargaining in higher education ". . . requires an exclusive agent . . ." and the educational units are generally represented by agents of the American Association of University Professors (AAUP), the American Federation of Teachers (AFT), or the National Education Association (NEA) (Baker, 1983, p. 781). Issues most generally negotiated, in addition to salary, include policies of appointment, reappointment, promotion, and tenure; teaching load, in terms of numbers of contact or credit hours assigned; fringe benefits; and organizational governance. Although collective bargaining is relatively unknown and very controversial among nursing faculties, it was present on nearly 700 college and university campuses in 1980 (Baker, 1983, p. 781), and it represents a growing trend. Nursing faculty and prospective faculty must become aware of the issues involved and prepare for involvement in the decision to unionize or not to unionize. Individuals seeking employment in unionized programs should learn the impact on employment considerations prior to signing the initial contract.

Politics in Educational Settings

Politics and the impact of political processes exist in educational settings as in all other major settings (Kalisch & Kalisch, 1982). Politics is often simplistically described as primarily a struggle for power. Others have identified a political situation as existing if, at any time, more than one individual desires or needs the same things.

Persons in educational institutions are many times engaged in unceasing struggles to gain recognition, honor, promotion, tenure, additional benefits, status, or academic freedom. Control of curriculum or roles in organizational decision making, and the processes, which influence and control all of these, are also highly contested political issues on campuses. There is little wonder that a unique political nature is inherent in all educational institutions.

Initially, it may be sufficient for a prospective or newly employed faculty member to know where policies and procedures relating to all faculty matters are housed and from whom interpretations and clarifications may be obtained. Sooner or later, it becomes important for each faculty member to know how to become involved in the politics of the organization. The organizational chart can be a clue if it is well developed and actually depicts how the organization is structured and by what mechanisms decisions are made. It is expected that deans accept responsibility for the successes, failures, decisions, and actions (or inactions) of the academic unit.

However, the *processes* by which advice, guidance, consultation, data, and other information are secured from the faculty are extremely important to the morale and well-being of faculty. Most faculties are organized around a faculty senate or assembly. The nature and responsibilities of such a body are crucial. At some institutions, senates have deteriorated into poorly attended conclaves given to meaningless oratory and little action. In such cases, the real power or decision-making activity is often in self-initiated special-interest groups of motivated, change-seeking faculty or core groups of change-resistant individuals. How much the faculty really know about how the decisions are made on salary, merit increases, tenure, nonreappointment, and workload may indicate clues about the power structure. The interactive and interdependent dynamics of a given educational unit indicate power sources.

In many instances, nursing faculty seem to believe that organizations make and will continue to make decisions about faculty, budget, facilities, and about other variables, which dictate quality of life. Some faculty believe these decisions are made through logical, rational, criterion-based processes that are stable over time. The politics of educational institutions and the nature of funding for those institutions (both public and private) render these assumptions naive. Financial or personnel decisions are often based on which group has the least power to resist, comprises the least influential constituency, and tends toward the least participation in university governance. It behooves nursing faculty, therefore, to learn to engage in the politics of the institution, increase the visibility of the nursing unit and its concerns, and initiate and maintain networks of support groups and organizations, which can be mobilized in a short period of time to help influence far-reaching decisions made at the institutional level.

RISKS

Risk factors inherent in positions in educational institutions are varied and can be important barriers to a successful life in academia. There are several risks regarding tenure, loss of clinical competence, professional liability, and grievances.

Tenure

Tenure is intended to provide security and academic freedom to those who attain it. The "up-or-out provisions" inherent in the process of achieving tenure, however, must be considered as a risk. The American Association of University Professors has endorsed seven years as the time limit for a probationary period for a faculty member. Most colleges and universities rigidly enforce this time limit for nontenured faculty in order to avoid issues of de facto tenure. De facto tenure may be best understood as tenure, which is neither earned nor awarded by the institution. It is a situation in which the rights and privileges of a tenured position are obtained by an individual by virtue of having been continuously employed full-time for a specified number of years.

For some faculty members, probationary periods are often fraught with such problems as self-doubt, anxiety over performance evaluations, and distrust of the process and the individuals who will ultimately make or influence the tenure decision. In addition, self-incrimination or guilt is common when well-made plans for educational advancement, publication, or research activities simply do not materialize. Some nontenured faculty liken the probationary period to an extended period in a glass house because every facet of behavior is closely scrutinized.

Tenure-eligible faculty must take risks, which involve decisions about where to concentrate available time, energy, and efforts. In a typical university system, demonstrable and frequent scholarly activities, involvement in professional activities and organizations, increasing excellence in classroom and clinical teaching, and community service activities are all demanded prior to final tenure review. The risk is greatest when a faculty member prepared with a master's degree is required to obtain a doctoral degree in addition to demonstrating competence in other areas of performance in the seven short years. Seven years seems like a long time when one first enters academia as a faculty member.

Some systems may not be as demanding as others. Major universities with graduate programs usually adhere strictly to doctoral requirements and research activities, while smaller colleges and universities or those with only baccalaureate programs *may* have slightly less rigorous requirements. Junior and community colleges may not require the doctoral degree, but may insist on a substantial number of years of experience in clinical settings and teaching. It is vitally important that each faculty member know and understand the tenure requirements and process at the employing institution.

The *risk* involved in attempting to earn tenure may be reduced by frequent and meaningful evaluation sessions with the chairperson or dean of the program. When it becomes apparent that all criteria for tenure *cannot* be met by an individual faculty member, the best course of action is to negotiate responsibilities that will result in the best possible letter of recommendation at the time of termination. Faculty who do not receive tenure should not feel that they are "failures," but hopefully, they can understand that there is simply more to accomplish in achieving tenure than time has allowed to be accomplished. Failure to understand or accept this fact may lead to frantic, ineffective efforts in all areas of the faculty role without a strong performance in any one.

Finally, tenure often results in an illusion of job security in academic settings, which may prove to be a risk. Individuals who aspire to tenured faculty positions believe that, once tenured, they are employed for life. It should be remembered that fiscal exigencies can cause universities to discontinue programs or close entire departments. Not even the AAUP guidelines mandate institutions to retain faculty when the program is discontinued.

Nursing programs have been especially vulnerable to attack in recent years. University administrations have moved to close nursing programs at such sites as Skidmore College and Duke University, and have attempted closures at Michigan State University and the University of Nebraska. Nursing programs are thought to be at risk because of the inordinately low faculty-to-student ratios in the nursing courses and the resulting high cost of student education. However, baccalaureate students generate tuition money from general education courses.

Faculty can minimize the risk of losing a position through program closing by learning what the institution has done with tenured faculty in other units in similar circumstances. Some institutions pride themselves with a record of *never* releasing a tenured faculty member. Others seem not to be so concerned. The individual faculty member can reduce the financial risk of such an occurrence by staying current in the content area of expertise and by striving continuously to improve and enhance the teaching–learning methods utilized. Then, if disaster strikes through program closure, a new position should not be difficult to obtain.

Loss of Clinical Competence

The loss of clinical competence is a problem of which all nursing faculty must be aware and must plan to avoid. Because nursing instructors must demonstrate to both students and to clinical agency associates the ability to deliver care as well as to teach the principles involved in the delivery of care, nursing faculty must devise methods of maintaining and increasing competency. In some schools, joint appointments can be negotiated. Some faculty who are employed on 9-month contracts work 1 or 2 months during the summer at an institution, which serves as a cooperating clinical facility. Faculty are sometimes able to maintain clinical expertise through military reserve activities. The importance of activities of this nature cannot be overemphasized. Although not explicit in tenure policies, lack of clinical expertise may lead to a negative tenure review.

Professional Liability

The probability of involvement in legal actions brought by injured patients or clients is just as high for faculty as for nurses employed in clinical settings. Faculty are at risk not only to be named in actions involving their own performance with patients and clients, but will also be named in any actions taken against students assigned to them. Many educational institutions provide insurance "coverage" for faculty; however, nurse faculty should have the limits of that coverage examined very carefully and augment it with professional liability policies when necessary. Generally, this is well worth the cost.

Faculty may also find that they need protection from legal action, which might be brought against them by a student or former student. Generally, these actions result from faculty awarding a student a failing or unsatisfactory grade or forwarding a recommendation for dismissal of a student on the grounds of drug abuse or conduct inconsistent with professional performance. These risks to faculty can be reduced by learning efficient methods of making anecdotal notes, becoming well-versed in institutional policies involving student grievances, and seeking early and definitive assistance from the chairperson or dean early in the situation. Also, personal liability insurance is useful as a protection while publishing in case of an unintentional failure to document work from other sources, for example.

Grievances

Sometimes faculty members are justified in filing a grievance against the institution where employed. There is generally a separate grievance policy available for faculty, which clearly delineates issues, which may be grieved, the steps to take, and the time frame under which the grievance must be lodged. The appropriate time to examine the policy is prior to the time it is necessary to use it. It may be wise for individuals to exhaust all informal means available to resolve the conflict or problem and then carefully evaluate the risk of filing a formal grievance against a colleague or employer. The individual should be aware that while the mechanics of filing a grievance may be simple, the politics of filing a grievance are complex. On the other hand, if the matter involves a serious violation of faculty rights, it should be pursued. Not to do so increases the risk of future disputes, inequities, lowered morale, and increased injustices.

Finally, are there risks to faculty who have vaulted the tenure barrier, found mechanisms to stay clinically competent, who engage in the political processes of the school sufficiently to insure ongoing input into the system, who are loved by students and colleagues alike? In truth, such an individual probably runs a tremendous risk of complacency and ultimate boredom. Unfortunately, burnout does not occur solely as a result of overwork, overcommitment. too much stress, and unmet expectations. Too long doing the same thing, teaching the same courses, or using the same clinical facility can result in faculty burnout of quite a different nature from the burnout described in current literature. Many tenured faculty experience decreasing challenges and insufficient stimulation, accompanied by a growing fear of moving, resettling, or changing positions. The positive attributes of tenure are somewhat offset by a growing reluctance, once it is obtained, to relinquish tenure and start out in a new system. The faculty member may become trapped in the system's security belt, which may tighten and constrict productivity and satisfaction.

RISK REDUCTION

General comments can be made about risk reduction and management. The individual at greatest risk in any discipline, including nursing education, is one who does not stay abreast of current trends, issues, and concerns of the discipline involved. How can an individual achieve this when circumstances prevent further education or extra time in clinical settings or extensive travel to workshops or institutes? A popular answer lies in the concept of "networking," which suggests a matrix or interlocking network of persons who will support and provide information, suggestions, and counsel for one another. This can work for personal needs, professional needs, or both. Networks can be important sources of noncritical feedback and may provide necessary information sharing, which leads to better decision making. Skills necessary for networking include establishing and maintaining communication and correctly evaluating relationships to determine "safe" supporters. Communication and evaluation, however, are tools of the trade for educators, and nurse educators often are able to use networking to good advantage.

The rewards available to nurses employed in educational settings have been discussed. Academic systems can bestow both material and intrinsic rewards.

Material rewards include moderate to good salaries, generally pleasant and comfortable work environments, reasonable plans for medical insurance and retirement benefits, and frequently, educational benefits for family members. Intrinsic rewards may include environments rich in intellectual stimuli, collegial support, professional and social recognition, flexibility in scheduling, support for further educational advancement, and freedom for expression of creativity. Faculty also enjoy access to programs, which promote intellectual and social well-being; opportunities to engage meaningfully in organizational governance; and the rewards, which come from bringing about change in the present by educating the practitioners of the future. Individuals who value such rewards would do well to explore a position in nursing education.

Risks are inherent in such positions. The notable risks include seeking after but failing to obtain tenure, erosion of clinical skills and relevance, involvement in legal suits unrelated to one's own clinical performance, and possibly falling prey to complacency and lost enthusiasm for addressing a challenge. If these risks do not outweigh the advantages of a teaching position, it should be possible to avoid or overcome them.

For every person aspiring to a position in education because it is an "easy job" or "part-time" position paying a full salary, a word of caution. Educational systems, as stated previously, do not exist for faculty members, nor do the goals of the institution relate directly to the goals of *individual* faculty. Very few, if any, faculty members are involved in less than a full-time commitment to the institution where they are employed. Although the scheduled contact hours may be less than 18 hours per week, the job expectations will rarely be accomplished in 40 hours per week. For most faculty, however, the joys and rewards of working in an environment supportive of the values that are most important to them far outweigh the risks involved in employment in an educational setting.

REFERENCES

American Association of Colleges of Nursing. (1986–1987). *Report on nursing faculty salaries.* Washington, D.C.

American Nurses' Association. (1985). *Facts about nursing 84–85*. Kansas City, Mo.: American Nurses' Association.

Baker, C. M. (1983). Faculty unionism: Issues and impact. In N. L. Chaska (Ed.). *The nursing profession: A time to speak.* New York: McGraw-Hill.

Kalisch, B. J., & Kalisch, P. A. (1982). *Politics of nursing.* Philadelphia: Lippincott.

Morris, V. C. (1981). *Deaning: Middle-management in academe.* Urbana and Chicago: University of Illinois Press.

Rosenfeld, P. (1987). Nursing education in crisis—A look at recruitment and retention. *Nursing & Health Care, 8*(5), 283–286.

8

Career Management

Margaret Denise Zanecchia, Ph.D., R.N.
and Carol A. Stephenson, Ed.D., R.N.

CAREERS

Faculty careers in any discipline of education demand the time and attention of the individual professional to properly manage. College-wide, approximately 500,000 full-time faculty and another 200,000 part-time faculty are actively pursuing an academic career (Bowen & Schuster, 1985, p. 1). It is anticipated another 400,000 to 500,000 new faculty appointments are needed over the next 25 years to replace the existing cohort.

With approximately 1400 collegiate nursing programs in the United States, careers for nurse educators account for a small percentage of these academic faculty positions. (American Nurses' Association, 1985, p. 152) If the average number of faculty in each nursing program was 25, then approximately 35,000 positions could exist. It is estimated at least one half of these replacement positions are needed by the year 2000.

Definition

The definition of a *career* implies lifelong commitment to a particular type of professional work or field of endeavor. A nursing career in higher education is one example. A career nurse educator is usually a full-time faculty member employed in an academic setting, i.e., a college or university. Career nurse educators also are employed in the hospital and community as in-service educational coordinators, and also as educational consultants or researchers in a variety of settings.

The Nurse Educator as a Professional Person

In 1957, Greenwood (p. 45) proposed five attributes, which distinguish a profession: systematic theory, authority, community sanction, ethical codes, and culture. After 30 years, these attributes continue to depict the nursing profession.

Professionalism in nursing is addressed in the ANA Code for Nurses. The statements of the code address qualifications; quality; informed judgment; competence, legal and ethical; a body of knowledge; and collaboration, to name a few. A code of ethics is considered an essential characteristic of a profession, as it provides a mechanism for standards review. The Code addresses certain career issues, which include: competence to practice, maintaining competence, continuing improvement, and maintaining conditions of employment (American Nurses' Association, 1976).

In a study involving nursing educators of diploma, associate-degree, baccalaureate-degree, and graduate programs, the educators were asked their attitudes on professionalism. The higher the educational preparation of the faculty, the higher the degree of professionalism was perceived. The components of professionalism were considered to be: professional organization, public service, self-regulation, autonomy, and a sense of calling to the field (Schriner & Harris, 1984). The nurse educator is first of all a professional person. A professional individual possesses essential values, attitudes, and personal qualities and has the essential professional education and clinical practice skills (American Association of Colleges of Nursing, 1986).

The Nurse Educator in the Scientific Community

The nurse educator is a member of a scientific community. Scientific activity includes dialogue, exchange, discovery, and questioning. Colleagueship is a mutual consulting relationship. This collaboration among nurse educators reinforces the scientific community (Fawcett, 1980).

The Nurse Educator as a Scholar

The nurse educator is an educated person, a scholar. Scholars are learned individuals who have acquired knowledge and educational talent, who demonstrate intellectual competence and excellent performance, and who exemplify creativity. A nursing scholar has been described as one who uses intellectual honesty to improve clinical competence. The scholar displays self-discipline and judgment and remains current in the discipline. Nurse scholars encourage inquiry and exemplify the highest academic, personal, and professional standards (Sams, 1976, p. 23).

The community of scholars refers to both the faculty and the students who study and discover together. Nurse educators, who are productive researchers, are demonstrating "scholarliness" and "community" when the research is shared with students and peers (Jacox, 1976, p. 31).

Students must be socialized by nurse educators to become scholarly practitioners. When adequately socialized, future professionals systematically inquire to find new relationships among clinical data (Schlotfeldt, 1985, p. 8). The new faculty also expects to be socialized and oriented to academia (Mills, 1983; MacPhail & Munro, 1983).

Orientation programs, a socialization environment, and support from role models are assisting mechanisms for novice faculty. The result of socialization is the achievement of a faculty identity reflecting a professional discipline (Mauksch, 1982).

FACULTY POSITIONS

Position Descriptions

Although most positions in nursing service have written position descriptions, including duties, the faculty in nursing education may not. Usually a position description is a major management tool. It communicates the responsibilities, specific duties, organizational relationships, authority delegations. and qualifications (Liebler, 1983). For the educator, the role and multiple responsibilities serve to describe the faculty position. Since a specific list of tasks or job analysis may not be available, some faculty may self-author a part of the description.

College administration utilizes the contracting letter, which states rank and usually departmental name. A reference is made to evaluation criteria contained in the faculty handbook or policy manual.

Titles and Categories of Positions

The title of the position may be synonymous with the rank in many institutions. Four categories, positions, and career titles exist in academic settings:

- Teaching staff
- Supporting staff
- Supervisory staff
- Administrative staff

Within each of the categories are various labels and titles (Table 8–1). But not all positions are found in every nursing program. Usually the size of the program and budget determine the number and type of supporting and supervisory staff.

TABLE 8-1. CATEGORIES OF POSITIONS AND TITLES

Category I: *Teaching Staff*
- Assistant instructor
- Laboratory instructor
- Clinical instructor
- Lecturer
- Adjunct clinical instructor
- Assistant, associate, and full professors
- Emeritus faculty
- Endowed faculty

Category II: *Support Staff*
- Recruitment faculty coordinator
- Clinical contracting faculty coordinator
- Media faculty coordinator
- Continuing-education faculty coordinator
- Grants faculty coordinator

Category III: *Supervisory Staff*
- Course coordinator (undergraduate, graduate, RN track)
- Level coordinator
- Division coordinator (upper–lower division)
- Chairman of department
- Program director

Category IV: *Administration of School*
- Assistant dean
- Associate dean
- Dean

Description of a Faculty Position

Faculty members are persons whose specific assignment is made for the purpose of conducting instruction, research, or public service as a principal activity (Fortunato & Waddell, 1981, p. 40). Usually, the position description of a nurse faculty member includes statements pertaining to:

- The number of contact hours per week
- The number of office hours per week
- The number of lecture hours per week
- The number of new lectures to develop
- The number of new student advisees
- The number of committee memberships

If these activities are not found in writing, verbal explanations should be made to the faculty (Carpenito & Duespohl, 1981, p. 19).

Position descriptions contain different types and time frames for assignments. Positions are related to the level of faculty rank. For example, a new faculty with the rank of assistant professor may not be expected to serve on as many major committees as one with higher rank. The requirements for membership on certain committees are that one must be a member of the faculty, employed at the college for a specific number of years.

The level or division coordinator role in nursing may in reality be one in which the faculty person is in between the dean and the other faculty. In some nursing schools, coordinators have decision-making power similar to that of the academic departmental chairperson, but usually this is not the case (Wakefield-Fisher, 1985). Following are examples of position descriptions for a course, level, and division coordinator.

Course Coordinator

Organizational Authority. Course Coordinators shall be appointed by the Dean of the School of Nursing with consultation from the Division Coordinators. Course Coordinators shall direct the implementation of a particular course, and shall report to the appropriate Division Coordinators.

Qualifications. Course Coordinators shall be faculty members who:

- Hold a full-time faculty appointment
- Are beyond the first year of service in the Division
- Have had at least two years of teaching experience in Baccalaureate nursing education

Responsibilities. In conjunction with the Division Coordinators, the Course Coordinators are responsible for providing educational leadership in interpreting and implementing the philosophy, purposes, and objectives of the undergraduate curriculum as they relate to the particular course. These responsibilities shall be carried out through such activities as (University of Massachusetts, 1978):

- Orientation of new faculty to the course
- Assignment of intra-course responsibilities to faculty, in conjunction with the Division Coordinator
- Coordination of the activities of the teaching team through regular meetings
- Coordination of and participation in the process of ongoing evaluation of the course and of the teaching effectiveness of individual faculty
- Carrying out the educational and academic policies and procedures of the University and the School of Nursing as they pertain to the particular course
- Coordination of the activities of the course with those of the program through regular meetings with the appropriate Division Coordinator

Level Coordinator

Each member of the level team is responsible to the coordinator, and the coordinator is responsible to the Associate Dean (University of Connecticut Personnel Policies, 1978).

I. Faculty development
   A. Is available as a sounding board for faculty frustrations and faculty guidance
   B. Keeps faculty apprised of professional meetings and workshops
II. Curriculum implementation
   A. Facilitates group functioning
      1. Keeps group moving toward predetermined goals
      2. Prepares an agenda and schedules team meetings
   B. Is the liaison with School of Nursing administration
   C. Coordinates activities to maintain the integrity of the established grid and objectives for the level and the objectives for each course
   D. Keeps appraised of student progress and provides follow-up as appropriate
III. Administrative function
   A. Has the authority for equitable allocation of responsibility among team members
   B. Plans with faculty member for coverage during faculty absences
   C. Plans for assignment of a liaison person to each clinical agency
   D. Coordinates the details of course implementation
      1. Orders for books and media
      2. Course outlines, handouts, reserve lists
      3. Laboratory assignments
      4. Submits grades to Registrar
   E. Consults with administration regarding recruitment needs and shares in the selection process
   F. Provides for orientation of new faculty to team
   G. Provides for student evaluation of each team member (both in classroom and clinical)
   H. Submits an annual evaluation report on each team member
   I. Serves on Dean's Advisory Committee
IV. Team member function
   A. Carries a reduced teaching load
   B. Participates in group decisions
   C. Represents the team in campus activities

Division Coordinator

Organizational Authority. Division Coordinators shall be appointed by the Director of the Division of Nursing to direct the implementation of the undergraduate program. There shall be a Coordinator for the Lower Division and a Coordinator for the Upper Division. Division Coordinators shall report to the Director.

The management of the Multimedia Laboratory shall be the responsibility of the Lower Division Coordinator.

Qualifications. The Division Coordinators shall be faculty members who:

- Hold professorial rank
- Are beyond the first year of service in the Division
- Have had at least two years of teaching experience in baccalaureate nursing education
- Have had experience as course coordinators
- Have had experience on either personnel or curriculum committees within baccalaureate nursing education

Responsibilities. In conjunction with the Director, Division Coordinators shall be responsible for providing educational leadership in the interpretation and implementation of the philosophy, purposes, and objectives of the undergraduate program. These responsibilities shall be carried out through such activities as the following (University of Massachusetts, 1978):

- For Faculty
    Orientation of new faculty to the Division of Nursing
    Assignment of faculty, in consultation with the Director and the Course Coordinators
    Coordination of activities of the teaching teams through regular meetings with the Course Coordinators
    Coordination and participation in the process of evaluation of teaching effectiveness
    Assistance in carrying out the educational and academic policies and procedures of the University and the Division of Nursing
- For Students
    Coordination of the academic counseling system
    Scheduling courses and clinical placements in consultation with Course Coordinators
    Coordination of the process of student evaluation of courses and teaching
    Maintenance of student records and reports as prescribed by the academic and educational policies and practices of the University and the Division of Nursing
    Meeting with students as needed to interpret or implement program philosophy, purposes, and objectives
- For Program
    Selection of clinical agencies appropriate to the objectives of the curriculum
    Assistance in maintenance of contractual arrangements with cooperating agencies
    Representing the Division of Nursing at appropriate interagency meetings
    Assistance in maintenance of program records and reports as prescribed in the educational and academic policies and procedures of the University and the Division of Nursing
    Coordination of program activities through regular meetings with the Director of the Division of Nursing

Nursing Faculty Member

The position description may include qualifications, functions, and responsibilities. A general description for a nurse-faculty member follows.

Qualifications. The nurse-faculty member shall be an experienced nurse and nurse educator who holds a Registered Professional Nurse License in the state, and shall possess the minimum degree of Master's for the undergraduate program and the minimum degree of Doctorate for the graduate program.

Functions and Responsibilities to the University

- Observe all University policies and regulations
- Serve as a member of the University Senate if elected by the School of Nursing faculty members and serve as a member of the University committees to which he or she may be appointed or elected
- Maintain mutually beneficial relationships with faculty from other disciplines in the University, colleagues in professional nursing outside the University, and individuals in the community
- Continually improve competence as a professional nurse, scholar, teacher, and citizen through formal and informal study, research, attendance at meetings, and participation in professional and educational organizations and in civic activities
- Observe the University calendar in relation to registration, vacations, examination week, and grade reports to the Registrar's Office
- Attend required University convocations in appropriate academic dress
- Hold a minimum of two office hours a week on campus and arrange to meet students by appointment at other times if requested by students.

Functions and Responsibilities to the School of Nursing

- Attend faculty meetings
- Assist the Division Director in fulfilling the mission of the Division and University
- Teach courses as assigned
    Accept the philosophy that his or her courses constitute an integral part of the total curriculum and that they should use and reinforce learning from preceding and concurrent core, prerequisite, and nursing courses
    Select objectives, course content, and learning experiences, which are consistent with the philosophy and objectives of the curriculum, and, which assist students to develop the competencies essential to the practice of professional nursing
    Develop, evaluate, and revise course outlines
    Create an environment in the classroom and community, which facilitates and encourages student learning
    Motivate and guide students to think, to question, and to critically analyze

Utilize a variety of techniques to evaluate student achievement and progress in terms of the course objectives
Serve as a professional role model for students
Send the signed student clinical evaluations to the Level Coordinator by the date of the final grade reports
- Report to the Program Chairman and Level Coordinator any problems of a serious nature, which may arise in relation to faculty, students, or the nursing program
- Carry out other assignments at the request of the Level Coordinator

Functions and Responsibilities to the Community Agencies

- Uphold the provisions of the University contract with the agency
- Communicate with the appropriate administrative official through a Level Coordinator
    Names of students
    Dates, times, and location of learning experiences
    Problems concerning student experience in the agency
- Wear appropriate attire in the agency—uniform or laboratory coat and name pin
- Orient students to the agency
    Introduce to agency staff
    Interpret agency policies and procedures
    Tour the physical setting of the agency
- Assume responsibility for the maintenance of student-staff relationships, which will facilitate student learning
- Assume responsibility for teaching, assigning, supervising, and evaluating students

Assistant Professor

A more complete description of the Assistant Professor position includes a title, qualifications, and professional experience. It describes contributions to student learning, the advancement of the profession, programs of the school, community service, and professional growth.

I. Academic Qualifications
   Minimum of Master's degree with appropriate clinical and educational specialization
II. Professional experience
   A. A minimum of two years' teaching experience at time of application
   B. A minimum of two years' clinical experience
III. Contribution to student learning
   A. Interacts appropriately and effectively with students
   B. Uses appropriate teaching strategies in classroom and clinical settings
   C. Designs a quality unit of instruction (objectives, content, examination items, and evaluation of the unit)

D. Organizes and presents classroom content in a manner that is logical to the students
E. Stimulates curiosity and thinking in students
F. Demonstrates command of the subject in classroom and clinical setting
G. Is objective and fair in evaluation
H. Serves as a role model for clinical nursing practice
IV. Contribution to the advancement of the profession
A. Participates in professional nursing organizations
B. Authors (or co-authors) articles, books, or chapters for publication
1. Designs (or co-designs) and implements a research project, or
2. Presents papers at professional meetings
V. Contribution to programs of the school
A. Participates in faculty meetings (committees, faculty organization) giving rationale for position on issues
B. Supports group decisions
C. Serves effectively as a member of at least one School of Nursing committee
D. Gives evidence of accepting and carrying out additional responsibility
E. Participates in identifying or interviewing potential faculty
F. Gives assistance to less experienced faculty members
VI. Contribution to community service
A. Participates in health-related community activities
B. Presents continuing education workshops in community workshops or clinical agencies in area of expertise
C. Assists in planning programs for the continuing education of nurses
VII. Professional growth
A. Participates in professional development programs
B. Takes academic course work related to nursing within past three years, or practices in an appropriate clinical area at least every three years with evaluation of practice

Associate Professor

The Associate Professor and Professor position descriptions include contributions to student learning for the Associate Professor, but other contributions are expanded at a high level (University of Texas, 1983).

I. Academic qualifications
An earned doctorate in nursing or a field allied to nursing
II. Professional experience
A minimum of four years' teaching experience in a Bachelor of Science in Nursing or Master of Science in Nursing program, at least two of which shall be in the School of Nursing
III. Contributions to student learning
A. Meets the criteria for Assistant Professor

B. Demonstrates attributes of a master teacher as evidenced by:
      1. Flexibility and innovation in instructional activities
      2. Maturity and composure in interpersonal relationships
      3. Diagnosing learning problems and intervening appropriately
      4. Enhancing student learning beyond prescribed course objectives
   C. Designs and implements a quality course of instruction
IV. Contribution to the advancement of the profession
   A. Participates in professional organizations
   B. Is sought as nurse educator consultant in areas of expertise
   C. Presents papers at professional meetings
   D. Authors (or co-authors) articles (in refereed journals), books, or chapters for publication, or
   E. Designs (or co-designs) and conducts a nationally known research project
V. Contribution to the programs of the school
   A. Meets the criteria for Assistant Professor
   B. Provides leadership on at least one School of Nursing committee
   C. Generates creative ideas to facilitate program development and implementation
   D. Serves as a consultant to peers
   E. Makes self available as consultant to administration
VI. Contribution to community service
   A. Meets the criteria for Assistant Professor (section VI of Assistant Professor description)
   B. Provides leadership in health-related community activities
   C. Contributes to the improvement of nursing practice
VII. Professional growth
   A. Maintains and improves clinical competency and scholarly endeavors through methods of individual professional development

Professor

I. Academic qualifications
   A. An earned doctorate in nursing or an allied field
II. Professional experience
   A. A minimum of seven years' teaching experience, at least five of which shall be at the baccalaureate or higher level; a minimum of two years at the School of Nursing as an Associate Professor
III. Contributions to student learning
   A. Meets the criteria for Associate Professor
IV. Contributions to advancement of the profession
   A. Provides leadership in professional organizations
   B. Serves as nurse educator consultant in area of expertise
   C. Presents papers at state or national meetings
   D. Authors (co-authors) articles (in refereed journals), books, or chapters

E. Designs and conducts ongoing research
   F. Recognized at local, national, or international level in area of expertise in nursing
V. Contributions to the programs of the school
   A. Meets the criteria for Associate Professor
   B. Acknowledged by students and faculty as a leader
   C. Formulates course of actions relative to issues influencing nursing practice or nursing education
   D. Offers constructive criticism and assistance relating to administrative decision making
VI. Contributions to community service
   Meets the criteria for Associate Professor
VII. Professional growth
   Meets the criteria for Associate Professor

Other Positions

Certain positions, which do not require advancement toward tenure, are special non-tenure-track positions. The qualifications are usually found within the practice area and expertise of the faculty applicant.

CHARACTERISTICS OF CAREER POSITIONS

Characteristics of careers in nursing education influence the faculty in the selection of faculty position. How much or how little growth potential there is in a career is highly correlated with career satisfaction, change, and mobility. In a study of nursing education, the satisfaction of the faculty was directly related to their degree of participation in decision making. Centralization was negatively associated with overall faculty satisfaction. The effect of centralization was most negative for faculty with the strongest desires for autonomy (Grandjean, Bonjean, & Aiken, 1982).

The organizational climate is another characteristic perceived by nursing faculty to make a difference in a career position. Feeling a team spirit and a sense of group goals in the program environment is more conducive to work by the faculty. An organizational setting of openness and trust is necessary to create a learning environment (Krampitz & Williams, 1983).

More professional autonomy is sought by professional nurse educators. Autonomy is an important characteristic for the faculty. Nursing faculty need to influence the public, other professionals, the lawmakers, and their peer colleagues on the campus (Van Ort, 1985, p. 234).

The importance of the leadership of the administrator or dean is an indicator of faculty satisfaction and retention. A dean who is perceived to be autocratic, paternalistic, or dictatorial in administrative style increases faculty mobility. Other position characteristics, i.e., salary, geographics, reputation of school, dean's leadership, and responsibility, can determine position selection. The reasons found to leave a position, i.e., salary, geographics, dean's leadership, workload, and academic freedom, are ranked in order of importance by Lenz and Waltz (1983).

The school's reputation is an important attractor of a nursing faculty to a position. The profile study of the top-ranked schools of nursing identifies quality program characteristics as determined by students, faculty, administrators, and community (Wandelt, Duffy, & Pollock, 1985). The 20 top-ranked schools of nursing were utilized, and a random sample of six schools were selected for study. The six schools were: the University of Washington (#1), the University of Illinois (#7), Wayne State University (#8), Catholic University of America (#9), the University of Maryland (#11), and Boston University (#13) (Chamings, 1984, pp. 238–239). The University of Texas at Austin (#14) was selected as the pilot.

Elements, which were thought to interact and constitute high-quality programs of nursing, were people, things, processes, and other elements. As perceived by the faculty, the characteristics of top-ranked school faculties included (Wandelt, Duffy, & Pollock, 1985):

- Expertise
- Diversity in clinical focus, educational background and experience, teaching strategies, research interests
- Commitment to students, the nursing care of patients, the profession, and research
- Flexibility and unity
- Respect, trust, collaboration, constructive competition
- Mutual support of senior faculty
- Freedom to disagree
- Communication of knowledge, speaking engagements
- Holding office in professional organizations at the national level
- Offering consultation

The reputation of a program is based on many criteria. There is no doubt faculty will desire a position in a program that enjoys a reputation for high quality. Characteristics of faculty and programs influence careers.

CAREER DEVELOPMENT

A career as a nurse educator realistically involves more than the students and the teaching. Time, energy, and a plan are necessary in career management for every faculty to accomplish all of the nonteaching responsibilities. In addition to the major roles of service and research, other duties arise. Governance and participatory management demand countless hours.

The question of why nurse educators choose to accept the increased demands and workload in academia and pursue a doctoral degree was addressed by Bauder (1982). Because they are nurses and many are women, they are socialized not to meet their own needs, but to nurture others and to be supportive and responsive.

Being the newer professionals in the academic institution, they want to demonstrate responsibility to the institutional mission and their male colleagues.

Depending on the university, faculty development through research and publication may overshadow teaching. When teaching, however, ranks as most important to a nursing program, the faculty strive for excellence in teaching. This decision results in little time for professional development, graduate study, research, and publication. Those who "do it all" can and do risk a burnout.

Sometimes due to the burnout and other reasons, faculty become career changers. Academic changers identify the deterrents to professional growth as (Herman, McArt, & Belle, 1983):

- Inadequate opportunities for career development
- Concern about future opportunities
- Role overload
- Insufficient support to develop grants
- Inadequate liaisons with research colleagues
- Barriers to interdisciplinary projects
- Lack of graduate students
- Not knowing resources for professional development available from their departments

Nursing career development implies that a nurse prepares herself or himself to assume a higher role than the one presently held. The career preparation for the nurse educator involves attaining the professional credentials, usually the terminal degree, and experience to perform the faculty role. Career development is a lifelong process, which can mean balancing personal and occupational goals through serious planning, creativity, and supportive significant others (Smith, 1982).

A career plan or profile is a self-assessment, which includes systematically establishing career goals. Identifying professional strengths and weaknesses is a part of the process. The plan should have a time table and short-term measurable objectives. Determining cost, resources, and support persons (mentors) are included. According to Bolles (1981), the world of work involves one from approximately 22 to 65 years of age. Forty-three years of life are available for the total career.

Professional Credentials

Faculty development is the process, which begins with the obtaining of professional credentials. Professional credentials of faculty members are classified as the possession of either or both (1) the appropriate terminal academic degree, usually the doctorate; and (2) the relevant and equivalent practical experience (Allen, 1949, p. 70).

The master's or doctorate degree and the practical experience (length of employment in nursing and teaching) of the faculty are expected to correlate with the positional rank and salary. Pursuing the doctoral degree for the career nurse educator in the college system is considered a must (Kelly, 1985, p. 332). Professional growth for faculty can also mean pursuing staff development, continuing education, leadership training, and competency-based career ladders in the clinical area of expertise.

Phases, stages, adjustments, and role changes take place in the pursuit of the doctoral degree. Correct timing and placement of the program in the life cycle of an individual are extremely important. Many personal and professional changes take place (Urbano & Jahns, 1986).

Role adjustments from employment status to new student environments are usually anxiety-producing. A mentor relationship with a doctoral faculty allows the student to interact as part of an adult-peer dyad. Opportunities for self-directed learning and problem solving are enhanced for the student with a mentor (Bolton, 1980).

Doctoral Education

Selecting a doctoral program for a career as a nurse educator is dependent on a number of factors. Future specialization, point in a career, prior graduate courses, particular needs, interests, location, cost, acceptance to the program, reputation of program, and family responsibilities affect the choice of program (Curran, Habeeb, & Sobol, 1981).

Doctoral programs and institutions chosen by nurse educators vary greatly. The Ph.D., Ed.D., D.N.Sc., and the N.D. are the most frequently sought doctorates. The prestige of the degree and the status of the institution often have some bearing on the quality rating of the nurse faculty candidate. Changes in prestige of institutions and programs and the time elapsed since the degree is earned are less important. The current ranking of prestige is important.

Having a doctorate implies achievement of the highest level of competence. The degree of the faculty should be relevant to the field of the subject matter taught. Often, little or no relationship exists between the subject matter studied in the doctoral degree program and the courses taught by the faculty. When the doctoral degree is non-nursing, the faculty member's master's degree is sought in the relevant field or area teaching assignment. Other doctoral degrees, i.e., honorary doctorates, degrees for sale, quasi-doctorates, and ABDs (all but the doctoral dissertation or final research project) are not usually a problem in nursing education as they are in other disciplines.

Doctoral programs in other areas than nursing supply faculty for many master's degrees and doctoral nursing programs. Until more nursing doctorate programs are made available, this may continue to be the case. Nurses with doctorates in areas such as educational psychology, higher educational administration, sociology, anthropology, rehabilitation, psychology, biology, and physiology can bring diversity to the nursing profession (Snyder-Halpern, 1984).

The choice of the type of doctoral degree depends on the individual's career goals. Whether research, theory, or educational administration is preferred, the program selected should have the essential emphasis needed.

Regard for the faculty positions as advertised is necessary. In a 1982 journal review of the educational credentials sought by potential employers, the doctorate was required for 36 percent and preferred in 58 percent of the graduate positions. Baccalaureate faculty positions required the doctorate for 6 percent of the positions, and in 56 percent of its positions the doctorate was preferred (Butts, Berger & Brooten, 1986).

Experience

Relevant experience may infrequently substitute for the earned terminal degree. Relevant experience means practical experience with the subject to be taught gained through expertise equivalent to an academic program. The assessment of experience for the renowned candidate is positive, while the unknown, less honored faculty candidate may not be able to qualify on the basis of experience without the terminal degree. A few exceptions exist.

Experience alone, unfortunately, is not sufficient preparation even for clinical teaching. Classroom and clinical teaching require the educational preparation of the terminal degree. The least experienced and the least prepared should not be assigned clinical instruction (Karuhije, 1986). In Karuhije's study, a majority of respondents stated their graduate education did not provide individuals with basic information on clinical instruction.

Continuing Education

Continuing education in the broadest sense is all additional education gained by the faculty to increase knowledge and skills. Professional career development incudes continuing education. Ensuring high-quality performance is believed possible through continuing education.

Types of Continuing Education

Informal Education. Attendance at conferences and meetings includes self-learning modules, interpersonal peer relationships, team teaching, "on-the-job" training, and journal clubs. Part-time employment and volunteer work done as a faculty member may also be continuing education. Serving on committees of the faculty and the community are also informal mechanisms for learning.

Formal Education. This includes courses, seminars, workshops, and programs in which continuing education units (CEUs) are earned and documented.

Subjects of Continuing Education. Although most nursing subjects meet the CEU criterion, some non-nursing subjects are needed by most potential nurse faculty. The preparation of a teacher should include: construction of the lesson, learning theory, teaching models, curriculum development, audiovisual production and accompaniment, speech, foundations, test construction, measurement, research, and computer literacy (Kadner, 1984). As the nurse educator advances in academic position, other career-related skills become increasingly important. These skills would apply to any discipline and involve many areas of human development (Breen, 1981, p. 9):

- Information management skills
- Design and planning skills
- Research and investigation skills
- Communication skills
- Human relations and interpersonal skills
- Critical thinking skills
- Management and administrative skills
- Valuing skills
- Personal development and learning skills

More recently, the business skills, grantsmanship, accounting, budget, writing reports, personnel, time management, resources development, audit, team building, and facilities planning have been emphasized. In addition, law and counseling skills are useful.

Upon joining the faculty, the individual nurse educator's responsibility for continuing educational development begins. The assessment of continuing education needs of the nursing faculty should commence on initial interview for every teaching position and continue with yearly conferences with the dean (Abruzzese, 1984).

Continuing to demonstrate expertise in the clinical area is the responsibility of the nurse faculty. Every two or three years, faculty are expected to practice nursing in their specialty area to remain proficient (Smith, Baasch, & Hoffman, 1984).

According to Abruzzese (1984), the areas of competence are clinical theory and practice, curriculum and learning, theories, nursing theories, teaching strategies, audiovisual equipment and resources, test construction, counseling students, clinical evaluation, group dynamics and group process, writing for publication, and research. She states, "Clinical practice needs are for practice one day a week or in the summer."

Others consider courses of study outside the nursing discipline not to be continuing education. Examples are education or psychology courses for higher non-nursing degrees. Those who prefer to count units of nursing content as continuing education have mandated nursing relicensure in some states accordingly.

The various states' licensing departments can advise the nurse educator on the number of CEUs necessary for renewal within the period of time mandated. In California, for example, 30 hours of continuing education in nursing must be documented and completed during each 2-year period to renew the professional nurse license (R.N.).

The CEU. A nationwide standard of measurement is acceptable practice: the CEU. The continuing education unit (CEU) is defined as 10 contact hours of participation in an organized continuing education experience under responsible sponsorship, capable direction, and quality instruction. Earnings can vary from 0.3 CEU to 2.5 CEU or more, depending upon the number of contact hours (Koltz, 1979, p. 41).

Resources. Resources for continuing education in nursing are numerous. Continuing education offerings are listed in a variety of current journals, newsletters of associations, local newspapers, and by university continuing education departments. Community health organizations, nursing (private) consultants, and business-based corporations also offer professional continuing education programs. The individual nurse educator may contact the state board of nursing for other resources.

Human resources development programs enhance the nurse educator's career potential. In the college setting. development programs can enhance recruiting efforts. Some higher education institutions have sophisticated training and development programs (Fortunato & Waddell, 1981). Some examples are:

- Time management
- Grantsmanship
- Writing skills
- Public relations
- New teaching techniques
- Stress management
- Preretirement counseling

Ongoing career development for faculty can be achieved through peer faculty activities within the individual's college or among other adjacent colleges. An endless array of expert teachers and subjects are available. In addition, time and expense are also advantageous to the planning. Nursing faculty bring a rich source of experience and education, which can be utilized for creative and innovative continuing education (Seigel, 1986).

Continuing education in nursing education is a mechanism to assist faculty in fulfilling the requirement for faculty accountability. The consumer movement expects the delivery of quality education by quality educators (Moore, Damewood, Floyd, & Jewell, 1984). Standards of care and standards of education necessitate lifelong learning for professionalism.

CAREER STRATEGIES

Retention of faculty will be enhanced through career advancement. Faculty development can include career guidance, rotating departmental chairpersons, leaves, tuition assistance, and time for graduate courses toward the doctorate.

Contemporary career management requires continuous nurturing. Nurturing strategies include establishing networks and mentorhoods. Also, preventing burnout is a priority career strategy for nursing faculty.

Networking

Networking has been described as the process of developing and using one's contacts for information, advice, and moral support (Welch, 1980). Linkages among nurse educators are viable resources, which stimulate and maintain the professional communication and support systems.

Networking is becoming more important as a career management strategy for nurse educators. Networking is basically an informational, support, and informal exchange process among individual faculty. Members of a network have the benefit of personal and professional contacts for support, feedback ideas, and subsequently referrals for positions.

However, networking imposes membership obligations on the nurse educator. Some of the responsibilities of the networker are maintaining contact and communication through telephone calls, letters, and conversation. Trusting relationships among those in the network are necessary. Networks change, and individual faculty enter and leave. New networkers must be continually cultivated on all levels: upward (chairpersons and deans), peer level faculty, and downward (the individuals to whom the faculty member provides support) (Puetz, 1983a, p. 51).

When the nurse educator sets up a network, the following groups may be considered as potential network members. The list is endless.

Potential Networks

- Current positions: nursing peers and administrators, university peers, administrators
- Past positions: peers and administrators of nursing schools
- Peers as classmates in graduate school
- Past graduate faculty
- Peer researchers, co-authors
- Friends, family, and relatives in the profession
- Other non-nursing faculty colleagues
- Peers and administrators of other college programs and in other institutions
- Nursing service
- Other professional and community association committee members
- Other members of local, regional, national, and international organizations
- Peer program participants
- Publishing peers
- Peer grant writers
- Peer project colleagues

Welch (1980, p. 147) recommends the inclusion of "stars" and "known doers" in a successful network. These network members require greater recruiting efforts.

Networking can be systematized through an exchange of business cards. When the nurse educator requests the card from others, individual faculty should also offer to exchange cards. Maintaining a current supply of business cards with correct name, title, credentials, address, and telephone number is essential (Puetz, 1983b, p. 14).

Networking is considered a vital and rewarding national movement for executive businesswomen (Spengler, 1982). Networking for professional nurses and nurse educators can be a successful strategy for careerists. Cooperative goals (not competitive) should be the focus of the network. Through networks, which share, trust, value, and support; members increase self-esteem, unity, and professional identity (Meisenhelder, 1980). The informal power derived from networking is an effective career survival strategy.

Mentoring

Mentoring is another strategy utilized by the nurse educator to enhance career development and career management. Faculty mentors are trusted counselors or guardians (Puetz, 1983a, p. 81). Mentors for nursing faculty are found performing many roles: counselor, exemplar, host, and sponsor. Counselors give advice, while exemplars are themselves role models. Hosts introduce and arrange, and sponsors share authorship (Puetz, 1983a, p. 90). The male business world has acclaimed its mentors in several cause–effect success stories.

The characteristics of the mentor's role in nursing education may involve indirect teaching and a caring relationship. A dynamic relationship exists between a "seasoned" faculty and the new protege. Preceptorships often lead to mentorships in academia.

The concept of a mentor is friend and colleague. According to Hamilton (1981), a mentor means different things. The fine criteria for a mentor were developed by Collins (1983). A mentor has a higher position than one mentored, is an authority in the field or area of expertise, is influential, is interested in the growth and development of the protege, and is willing to devote time and a caring commitment to the relationship. While the mentor may also be a role model, the difference between mentors and role models is that emotion in the relationship exists with mentors and is not existent in the role-model dyad.

As described by Vance (1982), a mentor is a teacher, sponsor, guide, patron, and advisor. Vance's study found that 83 percent of the 71 American nursing leaders had a mentor during the career development period and 93 percent of those mentored had been mentors to others.

The mentors of the influential nurses studied by Vance provided:

- Guidance for promotion
- Role modeling
- Intellectual stimulation
- Inspiration
- Teaching and tutoring
- Emotional support
- Financial advice

Mentors are particularly useful in career planning. Mentorhood can develop from the network of the faculty. One who has benefited from a mentor relationship should feel responsible to become a future mentor for another individual, and thus the cycle evolves and continues as a great benefit to the development of the profession.

The ideal mentor qualities include (May, Meleis, & Winstead-Fry, 1982):

- Compatible personal characteristics
- Confidence
- Competence
- Self-concept
- Respectable
- Willing to give of self
- Sincere interest in the protege

However, mentor–protege relationships are very individualistic. Qualities found in one mentor may not be those, which enable another protege to be as productive.

The importance of planned socialization of new faculty cannot be overemphasized. Mentors have been suggested as the agents to implement the orientation and academic socialization of new faculty (Megel, 1985). Survival in a career as nurse educator is impossible without appropriate socialization at the beginning. A mentor should be selected and assigned for this task.

In later developmental stages of mentoring, the faculty protege has a more collegial relationship with the mentor. A final stage involves the protege becoming a mentor for a neophyte faculty member. Mentorhoods exemplify collaborative efforts, which foster collegiality.

With regard to the development of scholarliness in the nurse educator, mentoring is essential. The ideal mentor situation is based on the mentor possessing education and experience in the specific area of the protege interest (May, Meleis, & Winstead-Fry, 1982). For example, if the protege is pursuing the development of clinical evaluation tools, the mentor would have a list of publications in this area.

The academic nursing dean can serve as a mentor for faculty. With a dean for a "coach" and a "teacher," faculty plan for a mentor-protege relationship, which uses a participant–observer method (Chamings & Brown, 1984). Some of the roles to observe in the dean as a mentor are leadership and administrative ability, sensitive communication and timing, budgeting, fundraising, political role, negotiating skills, research, time management, and the balancing of administration, teaching, and scholarship.

The practical benefits of mentoring are the helpful advice provided by caring, experienced faculty in the multiple roles of the nurse educator. However, some limitations of mentoring do exist. Potential problems may develop for the protege in the area of ownership of ideas and in the opportunity to express innovative ideas not mutually shared with the mentor (Megel, 1985).

Self-mentoring as a strategy was discussed in the literature (Darling, 1985, 1986). When suitable mentors are not available, resource finding, questioning and listening, reading and researching, taking a class, simply observing people, and simply "figuring things out" are some techniques the nurse educator may employ.

The idea of mentor matching or why some mentoring results in higher achievements for some and not for others has been questioned. The "goodness of the fit" between the mentor and the protege could depend on the stage of professional development of the protege, the past experience with authority, or the pattern of learning. These three variables can influence the effectiveness of the outcomes (Darling, 1985).

The literature varies greatly in the acceptable definition of a mentor and the nature of the mentoring relationship. Because of this inconsistency, the findings in mentor research have been questioned (Hagerty, 1986). More scholarly research is needed to discover if mentorship is the approach for the successful development of the nurse educator career as an independent creative self-initiator. However helpful, mentored nurses are more likely to become mentors for others later in their careers.

Preventing Burnout

Lack of mutual psychological, personal, and professional support among nursing educators may lead to job stress and burnout. If the nursing profession provided support and leadership, role modeling, and mentoring, perhaps less burnout would occur in academia.

Burnout is a potential problem for nursing faculty, involving many consequences of job stress. However, burnout is defined as a syndrome that includes physical, emotional, and mental fatigue, feelings of helplessness and hopelessness, and lack of interest or enthusiasm for work and life in general (Muldary, 1983, p. 10). Because burnout is prevalent in the helping professions, nursing faculty as providers of humanistic services (teaching and peer relationships) are particularly vulnerable to burnout.

Four levels of stress exist prior to the state of burnout (Frain & Valiga, 1979). Applied to the nursing faculty, the levels include:

Stress Level	Symptoms
Level I	Includes day-to-day routine events, faculty not generally aware.
Level II	Faculty is aware of stress demand, may take action.
Level III	Faculty commences emergency behaviors.
Level IV	Faculty unable to deal with stressor—burnout occurs

Symptoms of burnout can include signs of poor physical health, weight gain or loss, alcohol and drug usage, depression, low life satisfaction and motivation, and absenteeism. Other signs of burnout are loss of concern and respect for oneself and one's peers, low creativity and low effective problem-solving ability, low morale, and negative attitudes (Ray, 1984). Faculty may spend less and less time with students and avoid peer faculty.

Faculty burnout symptoms are similar for nurse educators and others who teach. Disengagement from teaching duties or activities and from contact with students, detachment from previous peer relationships, and loss of spirit, ideals, and energy are signs of faculty burnout.

Because burnout is related to job stress, coping abilities in the burned-out faculty may be inappropriate or ineffective. As nursing faculty are members of the health professions, health care can be indirectly affected through the faculty, who may not be able to perform efficiently.

Recognition of potential burnout in nurse educators is an important strategy. The proposed five stages of Veninga and Spradley (1981) are helpful to diagnosing burnout:

- Honeymoon
- Fuel shortage
- Chronic symptoms
- Crisis
- Hitting the wall

Burnout potential for nursing faculty may be increased because of the increased responsibility. A relatively small group of educators must upgrade the profession and the quality of nursing. The escalating of the need for theory development in nursing as a practice base is a great commitment.

Role overload in nursing education accounts for much stress, which can lead to burnout. The pressure for faculty practice and publication productivity are major stressors (Wakefield-Fisher, 1983). No individual can fulfill all role expectations simultaneously. The environmental stress of being responsible for the care of many students and many patients in the clinical area is demanding. In addition, the monotony of grading numerous papers and care plans leads to overload (Jeglin-Mendez, 1982).

Nursing faculty may experience burnout due to administrative pressures to retain faculty who risk displeasing the student (appeal) and the administration because of a decision involving student failure and dismissal. Even more distressful is having the decision reversed by the dean, which can cause the preliminary hopelessness of burnout.

The newer student consumers of the baccalaureate or graduate degree in nursing are changing from the typical generic student to the R.N., first-time adult learner, career changers, homemakers, or transfer students. The new student can and does demand more time and higher grades for less quality work from faculty than in previous years. Advising, remedial work, counseling, and coaching mean added pressure for faculty's already time-ladened schedule and the potential burnout state (Lenhart, 1980).

Self-identified stressors of nursing faculty found in the role were related to four areas (Hinds, Burgess, Leon, McCormick, & Svetich, 1985):

- Academia, i.e., managing time and research
- Administration, i.e., dealing with politics, power, incompetent faculty
- Clinical, i.e., objective evaluation
- Classroom, i.e., innovative test methods construction

Job-related stressors influence the ability of the faculty to perform the role successfully. A degree of difference in levels of stress may exist between tenured and not-yet-tenured faculty. Some nursing faculty may attempt to engage in all of the roles simultaneously, causing self-burnout (Farabaugh, 1984).

Preventive strategies for faculty to employ in burnout are desirable: for example, the control of one's workload with rotations and substitutions. Support from the dean and administration is necessary. Faculty who are involved in policy formation and decision making will be less likely to burn out. Interpersonal relationships with support persons, especially peers, can serve as a sounding board for stress signs. Increasing rewards for the service will be effective prevention. Discharging tension through regular exercise while building inner psychological and emotional strengths can be done on an individual level.

CAREER GOALS

Faculty Evaluation

Evaluation is a major consideration in the career of any university or college faculty member. In order to progress in the academic system, the faculty member must be prepared to be evaluated at least once a year and perhaps more often.

Many young faculty members (and some older ones) are threatened by the evaluation process. In theory, at least, this should not be the case. Evaluation can be a useful process to the faculty member as well as to the institution. It is a way for the faculty member to take stock of what has been produced, to get some positive feedback for accomplishments, and to restructure goals and activities for the future. It is the method by which the chairperson, dean, president, or other decision-making group gains data for the purpose of making salary, promotion, retention, and tenure decisions.

An understanding of the academic evaluation process is helpful. However, the process is often not uniform or clearly delineated (Bobbitt, 1985). This may lead to the confusion and frustration of the person who is being evaluated. The best-working evaluation process is one which has a systematic plan, clearly delineated criteria and types of data to be submitted, and in which deadlines for submission are clearly stated well in advance. Each institution has the privilege of developing its own evaluation process. Within that framework, individual departments may further define the process and criteria specific for that department. Ideally, these criteria and evaluation tools are developed by the faculty themselves. Faculty participation will decrease the threat of evaluation and stimulate more cooperation in the process.

The Process of Evaluation. As previously stated, all institutions are different, but some practices are typical. The process in a typical university may commence with hiring. Early in the academic year or soon after the time of hiring, the dean or chairperson clearly explains the evaluation process to faculty and provides them with any forms and guidelines, which have been developed. Individual interviews with faculty members may be held for the purpose of discussing goals for the year and possibly for negotiating weighting of accomplishments. The faculty evaluation usually involves the areas of teaching, research, publications, and community service. It is unlikely that any one person can excel in all four areas each year. Therefore, many academic institutions provide for negotiation so that the faculty member can concentrate on two or three of the areas. Since teaching is the reason for the existence of the university or college, it is usually included as one of the priority goals (Bobbitt, 1985).

The pre-evaluation interview also serves to alert the dean or chairperson regarding the faculty member's interests and goals for the coming year. The dean can gain feedback on goals that seem inappropriate or creative ways to meet goals. If the faculty member then needs relief time for related conferences, courses, or other support, the dean who is aware of individual needs is more likely to provide that support. When necessary, the dean or chairperson can work to distribute workloads to allow faculty to achieve goals. This is often a problem in nursing departments because standard university workload formulas do not allow for the large number of hours necessary for clinical teaching.

The faculty member then finalizes goals for the coming year. Often an interim conference with the dean is held to check progress. When evaluation time is scheduled, the faculty member collects as much data as possible from as many sources as possible and prepares a packet or report using the format specified by the institution. The faculty member should systematically collect data throughout the year regarding activities and accomplishments. An easy way to do this is to have one specific folder in a desk drawer into which supporting data, programs from continuing education experiences, etc., can be filed until time to prepare the report. Once the report is prepared, it is evaluated by the chairperson or dean and possibly by the department or university tenured faculty committee and the university administration.

Evaluation Content. The content of the evaluation is usually in the four previously stated areas: teaching, research, publications, and service to the university and the community. There are several critical things for the faculty member to know about evaluation content very soon after employment: How are data to be secured? Does the faculty member do it independently, or are there specific forms and procedures? What evidence is considered most valuable? What type of evidence is required to support participation in community and continuing education activities? Is the faculty member expected to get letters from agencies? If so, are confidential letters considered better than nonconfidential? How do faculty usually secure peer input within the department? Is one form of organizing the review folder considered better than another?

Evaluation Criteria. The criteria for each area of the evaluation may or may not be clearly stated, depending on the institution. Hopefully, there are at least a job description and some general criteria. If such criteria exist, the faculty member should be certain to address these clearly in the report.

If there are not clear criteria, or areas that are important are not covered in the format, these can be added. For nursing faculty, one area, which must often be added is the issue of maintaining clinical competence. As yet, many academic institutions do not have criteria to recognize the time, which is spent maintaining clinical competence in nursing. Most nursing faculty agree that clinical competence is important, but it is difficult to find time to maintain competence when there is already a full workload. Indeed, some universities have rules against accepting outside employment. This reduces the faculty member to clinical practice only during the summer, if it is allowed then. This presents a paradox: "On one hand the system advocates the teaching of up-to-date knowledge, the researching of relevant nursing problems, and the writing of current and innovative nursing publications [while limiting] access to the real world'' (Porth, 1978). The faculty member may be able to negotiate a joint appointment with a clinical agency in order to maintain clinical competence or may be able to conduct clinical research or write clinically related articles in order to demonstrate competence. It is the opinion of this writer, however, that it is highly unlikely that writing articles or conducting research will be adequate to maintain clinical competence.

Evaluation Outcomes. Once the report is submitted and reviewed, an evaluative statement, which also includes recommendations regarding salary, promotion, retention, or tenure, is written. Authorship of this report varies from institution to institution. The faculty member should receive a copy of this report and have an interview with the dean or chairperson regarding it. Faculty should also have access to a well-specified grievance procedure if there is any disagreement with the report. This grievance procedure should be followed calmly and courteously. This is not the place or time for threats, legal proceedings, or the like. A positive outcome of the evaluation process is self-satisfaction for the job, which has been accomplished during the year. It can also generate ideas for self-improvement during the coming year.

Data to Be Included in an Evaluation Report. Self-evaluation is clearly an essential part of the report. Agency format should be followed if it is available. In general, a self-evaluation might include an updated vita, a list of courses, which have been taught; a list of other activities, which have been carried out for the college (such as advising and committee work); activities, which have been carried out for the university (such as university committees or serving as a marshal for graduation exercises); research, which has been completed or is in progress (with copies as available); publications or recently submitted articles; and a list of community service activities.

In paragraph form, the faculty member should discuss the year's activities in each of the four major areas: teaching, service, publications, and research. Any particular accomplishments or innovations in an area should be discussed, as should any problems, which arose and were creatively solved. In addition, the self-evaluation report should list the goals, which were determined for the year and discuss how they were met or why they were not. Evidence of meeting the goals could be included (such as a copy of an article or a project). There should be new goals stated for the coming year, though these may ultimately need to be negotiated with the dean or chairperson. When stating goals, it is critical to remember that the faculty member will tend to receive a more favorable evaluation if he or she works on goals, which are considered important by his administrator, rather than goals, which may be personally important but are considered unimportant by administration. Another useful area to include in the self-evaluation report is a summary of strengths and weaknesses and areas of growth during the past year (Fig. 8–1).

Directions:
Due Date:
Prepare a self-evaluation report, which contains the information listed below. In your discussion of each area, list your goals, which you set for the year. Present evidence of achievement of each goal by discussion or attached materials. Cite additional achievements, which are pertinent in any area. Discussion should cover the academic year, which is closing at the time of this report.

Sections for Self-evaluation Report
1. **Teaching.** Include here your assessment of any changes or improvements you have made in your classroom and clinical teaching and in advising during the year. Please highlight those changes you decided to make to improve or enhance your own skill as a teacher, as opposed to those made because of curricular changes or team decisions. You may attach anything you wish to illustrate your activities-revised syllabi, description of a new teaching technique, a new evaluation procedure, a new procedure for advising, etc.
2. **Publications.** Include articles, chapters, books published or in press.
3. **Research.** Include current or completed research.
4. **Service.** Describe service to the community and to professional groups (such as being a board member for the heart association).
5. **Other professional activities.** List speeches or papers presented, workshops conducted, activity to maintain clinical competence, and others.
6. **Participation in team work.** Include a description of responsibilities you have had as a team member or team leader during the past year and activities you undertook voluntarily to enhance the effectiveness of the team as opposed to your normal work assignment. However, if in your opinion, you assumed more than the normal amount of teaching, planning, or clerical work of the team, you should certainly describe your workload.
7. **Contributions to the school or university.** Include committee memberships, responsibilities within committees; chairmanship; special assignments; other services you may have been asked to perform or volunteered to perform, etc.
8. **Professional growth (self-improvement).** Include courses taken, workshops attended, professional conventions attended, individually designed growth activities, professional groups, memberships, etc. Describe level of activity in professional organizations.
9. **Achievement of goals for the past year.** List goals as set forth at the beginning of the year or in last year's report. Discuss how each was met or what activities were carried out toward meeting a goal. If a goal was not met, briefly explain.
10. **Specific professional goals for the coming year** in each of the areas described above along with possible activities designed to fulfill the goals. Try to be as specific and realistic as possible, since these goals will form the basis for the next self-evaluation report (Stephenson, 1980b).

Figure 8–1. Sample guidelines for faculty self-evaluation report. *(Figures 8–1 through 8–6 adapted from materials developed by the Affairs Committee, C. Stephenson Chairperson, Baylor University School of Nursing, 1980a–f . Fig. 8–1 from Stephenson, 1980b.)*

Peer evaluation should also be a part of the report. Faculty peers should evaluate performance in the classroom and in collegial activities such as committee work. The best way to obtain these evaluations is to request that trusted faculty colleagues attend some classes and complete a form regarding the class presentation (Figs. 8–2 and 8–3).

Faculty _____ Team or Committee _____
Term _____ Evaluation _____

Directions: Please complete the following as objectively as possible. Your additional comments will be appreciated.

Rating Scale:	Consistently Demonstrated		Average		Never Demon.	Not Applicable
	1	2	3	4	5	X

Personal characteristics   COMMENTS:
_____ Demonstrates flexibility
_____ Displays a sense of humor appropriate to the situation
_____ Displays enthusiasm
_____ Listens actively and openly

Interaction with others
_____ Sensitive to other's feelings
_____ Facilitates exchange of ideas
_____ Solicits and respects others point of view
_____ Recognizes accomplishments and strengths and potential of others
_____ Recognizes and accepts individual differences

Professionalism
_____ Works to increase own professional growth
_____ Maintains professional relationships with others
_____ Identifies own strengths and limitations
_____ Uses meeting times effectively and for task resolution
_____ Takes responsibility for own actions and decisions
_____ Is a positive role model, professionally and personally
_____ Is motivated and motivates others

Expertise
_____ Is informed of advances in area of specialty
_____ Is prepared for the educational setting
_____ Utilizes appropriate facts, concepts and principles related to both education and nursing

---

Figure 8–2. Sample peer evaluation of committee work (*from Stephenson, 1980f*).

```
Faculty _____ Visitor _____
No. hours class evaluated _____ Course _____ Term _____

Rating      Consistently          Average              Never      Not Appli-
Scale:      Demonstrated                               Demon.     cable
                 1        2          3        4          5          X
```

Organization and planning
_____ Class presentation well planned and organized
_____ Major class objectives emphasized and made clear
_____ Lecture relevant to objectives
_____ Class time well used
_____ Provided appropriate closure

Mastery of content
_____ Has mastery of content, including current advances
_____ Recognizes own limitations and handles these appropriately

Level of thinking
_____ Encourages critical thinking and analysis
_____ Teaches for transfer and application of learning

Clarity of presentation
_____ Important ideas explained clearly and at the appropriate level of understanding
_____ Class is interesting
_____ Voice and mannerisms appropriate
_____ Audiovisual aids used appropriately and skillfully
_____ Uses appropriate teaching techniques

Climate and interactions
_____ Teacher's attitude toward the subject is enthusiastic
_____ Confident and at ease
_____ Demonstrates flexibility
_____ Demonstrates enthusiasm
_____ Good attitude of class toward teacher
_____ Reacted appropriately to questions
_____ Reacted appropriately to viewpoints different from his or her own

COMMENTS

Figure 8–3. Sample classroom visitation appraisal (*from Stephenson, 1980a*).

The peer who evaluates the class should be honest and should be careful to point out strengths as well as weaknesses. The form is submitted to the faculty who taught the class, who reviews it and includes it in the evaluation packet. If there are specific suggestions for improvement, comments to address the suggestions may be included in the narrative. If there is time before the report is due, work on overcoming the weaknesses may be accomplished and peers invited back to do another evaluation. Both evaluations would then be included in the packet. Peer evaluations should also be done regarding committee work. Again, having a specific form for this purpose is extremely helpful (Fig. 8–2). Usually, the faculty asks committee chairmen to write this type of evaluation.

Chairperson Evaluation. The person to whom the faculty member reports directly should visit the class for evaluative purposes at least yearly. If they exist in a particular institution, middle managers such as team or level chairpersons would do this evaluation. If the faculty member reports directly to the dean and there is no middle manager, the dean should visit the classes. If the faculty teaches both theory and clinical courses, both courses should be visited. The visitor should talk with students as well as observing faculty and should complete specified evaluation forms.

Student Evaluation. There is a wide divergence of opinion regarding the value of student evaluations. Most schools request that they be obtained, though some place a much higher value on them than do others. Some faculty feel that this evaluation reflects on the student as much as on the teacher. Not all students wish to participate in faculty evaluation (Bobbitt, 1985), which may present a problem in getting a representative sample of student evaluations. Timing is important, both in getting students to do evaluations and in what the evaluations will say. Handing out the evaluation forms just after a difficult examination or after clinical evaluation conferences may result in students not completing the form or in students venting their frustrations on the evaluation. It is often helpful to give out the evaluation forms during the last class period before the final examination in the course, or in a clinical course, having the forms completed before the final clinical evaluation conference. A neutral person should collect and tabulate the evaluation results (Sullivan, 1985) (Figs. 8–4, 8–5, and 8–6).

In a report, which includes student evaluations, use of evaluations over a course of several semesters or years is much more informative than evaluations for one semester or year alone. This can be done with tables or graphs to compare composite evaluation scores for each semester or year. If the university uses computerized evaluations and average scores for the department faculty and they are available, these can also be plotted against the individual faculty member's scores. This is especially helpful when the faculty is receiving scores above the college average or when the evaluations are moving closer to the college average.

Agency Evaluation. If the faculty member is teaching clinical courses, it is helpful to secure letters from several agency personnel (such as head nurses or charge nurses) with whom the faculty has worked closely. The letters can be brief, but should address such issues as how the faculty member represents the university, his or her work with students, role modeling, and how the faculty interacts with staff. Agency personnel should be encouraged to be open and frank in these evaluative letters.

```
┌─────────────────────────────────────────────────────────────────────┐
│ Faculty _____ Academic Year _____    │
│ Rotation _____ GPA _____ Level of Student _____   │
│ Directions: Please rate your clinical instructor in each of the major areas listed below. │
│             Your comments and suggestions will be appreciated.      │
│ Rating     Consistently        Average         Never    Not Applicable │
│ Scale:     Demonstrated                        Demon.                │
│                 1          2        3      4     5          X       │
├─────────────────────────────────────────────────────────────────────┤
│                                            COMMENTS                 │
│ _____ Sets realistic goals for or with the                        │
│         student                                                     │
│ _____ Facilitates the use of appropriate expe-                    │
│         riences to meet clinical objectives                         │
│ _____ Helps in new situations without taking                      │
│         over                                                        │
│ _____ Is available to the student as a re-                        │
│         source person                                               │
│ _____ Encourages student to think for himself                     │
│ _____ Relates classroom theory to clinical                        │
│         situations                                                  │
│ _____ Provides appropriate constructive feed-                     │
│         back while student is performing in the                     │
│         clinical area                                               │
│ _____ Provides constructive feedback on writ-                     │
│         ten assignments                                             │
│ _____ Demonstrates skill in nursing activities                    │
│         when required                                               │
│ _____ Contributes to an atmosphere which is                       │
│         conducive to student learning                               │
│ _____ Promotes learning through the ex-                           │
│         change of ideas in group conferences                        │
│ _____ Demonstrates understanding and rec-                         │
│         ognition of the individuality of the                        │
│         student                                                     │
│ _____ Evaluation of performance is objective                      │
│         and constructive                                            │
│ _____ Is a good professional role model                           │
└─────────────────────────────────────────────────────────────────────┘
```

Figure 8-4. Sample opinionnaire regarding clinical instructor (*from Stephenson, 1980e*).

Other Supporting Data. Other data, which can be helpful are letters from community agencies documenting community service, thank you notes from students and others who received services from the faculty member, programs from workshops attended, certificates awarded, and the like.

Organizing the Report. If the institution specifies a format for the report, it should be carefully followed. The report should be neatly typed without misspellings or major flaws. It should be organized so that each document is clear as to what it is

| Faculty _____ | Academic Year _____ |
| Course _____ | GPA _____ |

Directions: Please rate your classroom instructor in each of the major areas listed below. Your comments and suggestions will be appreciated.

Rating Scale:	Consistently Demonstrated		Average		Never Demon.	Not Applicable
	1	2	3	4	5	X

COMMENTS

_____ Contributes to an atmosphere which promotes learning

_____ Appears to demonstrate comprehensive knowledge of subject matter

_____ Presents content which meets the class objectives

_____ Presents subject matter in an organized manner and at an appropriate level

_____ Emphasizes the most significant concepts

_____ Demonstrates ability to ask thought-provoking questions

_____ Is open to questions from students

_____ Answers questions clearly and concisely

_____ Utilizes appropriate examples and audiovisual aids to demonstrate conceptual and clinical applications

_____ Clarifies material which requires elaboration

_____ Speaks effectively (clarity, eye contact, loudness, poise)

_____ Demonstrates involvement in and enthusiasm for content

_____ Stimulates your interest in subject matter

_____ Facilitates your overall learning of the subject matter

Figure 8–5. Sample opinionnaire regarding classroom instructor (*from Stephenson, 1980d*).

| Faculty _____ | Academic Year _____ |

Directions: Please rate your advisor in each of the areas listed below. Your comments will be appreciated.

Rating Scale:	Consistently Demonstrated		Average		Never Demon.	Not Applicable
	1	2	3	4	5	X

Professional role model
_____ Is expert role model for both theory and clinical roles
_____ Demonstrates professional and interpersonal skills articulately

Student advocate
_____ Facilitates progress of individual student as indicated
_____ Is sensitive to indicators of student need

Information giving
_____ Information given is accurate
_____ Refers student to appropriate resources, persons, materials

Information seeking
_____ Assesses individual needs and tries to meet these needs appropriately
_____ Protects privacy and confidentiality

Encouragement
_____ Gives constructive and helpful criticism
_____ Displays genuine interest in student

Facilitates problem solving
_____ Assists in defining the problem
_____ Assists rather than imposes problem-solving
_____ Is supportive of student's solutions to problems
_____ Appropriate referrals

Coordinating
_____ Assists appropriately in adjustment to campus, coordination of activities

Academic advisement
_____ Monitors and counsels academic performance appropriately
_____ Encourages and facilitates the development of special interests

Other personal characteristics
_____ Is approachable
_____ Is available
_____ Is reliable

COMMENTS

Figure 8–6. Sample opinionnaire regarding academic advisor (*from Stephenson, 1980c*).

and where it fits in the report. If no particular format is specified, a nice way to do it is with a loose-leaf notebook. The faculty member can use dividers to separate out different parts of the report such as self-evaluation, student evaluations, lists and copies of publications, etc.

Tenure

Definition. Although tenure is somewhat controversial today, nearly every university has a tenure system. It is critical that the new faculty member have some understanding of that system. According to the American Association of University Professors (AAUP), tenure "is an arrangement under which faculty appointments in an institution of higher education are continued until retirement for age or disability, subject to dismissal for adequate cause or unavoidable termination on the account of financial exigency or change in institutional status" (American Association of University Professors, 1975).

Advantages and Disadvantages of Tenure. The main purpose of tenure "is to insure academic freedom and provide sufficient economic security . . ." (Farmer, 1976). This means that once tenure is achieved, the faculty member can have academic freedom to teach as he or she wishes (within reason) without fear of losing the job because those inside or outside of the university disagree with the teaching. Tenure may be lost if there is an extremely major problem with the faculty's individual conduct. The advantages of tenure, therefore, relate to job security and academic freedom.

There are some disadvantages to tenure. If the university is not careful, a large proportion of faculty could be tenured, and this will limit the number of new persons who could be hired. This could limit the flow of new ideas and intellectual growth. Having large numbers of tenured faculty also limits faculty mobility and reduces job opportunities for newly qualified faculty.

One method of dealing with the tenure problem, which is currently used in some universities, is the creation of a nontenure track in addition to the tenure track. Those who hold master's degrees or are otherwise not in a position to seek tenure can be hired into the nontenure-track positions. Longevity in these positions varies greatly from school to school. Some institutions limit the employment of nontenure-track faculty to only five years; others require that nontenure-track faculty work only part-time. Some institutions give nontenure-track faculty full-time one-year appointments, which are subject to review each year.

Tenure Criteria. Tenure criteria have changed a great deal in the past years as universities attempt to limit the amount of persons receiving tenure and thus not overload the university with tenured individuals. As a part of the university, the nursing department must meet university standards for tenured faculty. Currently, tenure eligibility usually requires an earned doctorate along with publications and research. In some institutions, achievement of associate professor status is also a requirement. In other schools, appointment as associate professor comes along with the tenure decision. In some instances, a newly hired dean is granted tenure at the time of hiring. This does not tenure the person in the dean's position, but as a faculty member only. In still other institutions, rank and tenure are unrelated. In general, tenure criteria should be clearly stated and available to the faculty member from the time of employment. The criteria need to be flexible enough to allow for varying faculty roles (Bobbitt, 1985). Meeting the criteria for tenure may be a problem for nursing, as stated earlier, due to the heavy faculty loads caused by clinical courses and by lack of acknowledgement for the time and effort spent in maintaining clinical competence.

The university should have stated criteria for tenure. These criteria usually relate to quantity, quality, or potential accomplishments. Potential accomplishments are the most difficult to measure and often receive the least weight if they are considered at all (Porth, 1978). Quantity refers to the number of works, products, services, or whatever else the faculty member has accomplished. Quality is considered variously by different schools. For example, publishing in refereed journals may be considered superior to publishing in nonrefereed journals. Publications are usually considered superior to speeches and presentations. Institutions view single-author publications differently from multiple-author publications. Some institutions view every publication equally, even if a given faculty member's name is last in a long series on every one of his or her publications. Others give more credence to single-author publications. The faculty member would do well to know the stance of administration at the particular institution regarding the interpretation of tenure criteria.

When to Seek Tenure. When a faculty member is hired at a university, there should be probationary or get-acquainted time. This is usually 3 to 7 years. At the end of the stated period, the faculty member is either tenured or receives a terminal contract for 1 year. After that terminal year, employment must be sought elsewhere. The date of tenure review is usually stated at the time of employment. Experienced faculty members are allowed to "bring in" time to reduce the seven years commonly required for tenure. Often, the faculty member is allowed to negotiate the number of years to be brought in. In order to negotiate a manageable number of years, the new faculty member should look closely at the institution's tenure criteria. Can all that needs to be accomplished be done in the number of years allowed (example: competent teaching, publications, research, etc.)? If the new faculty member has few accomplishments in these areas, probably all 7 years are needed to get ready for the tenure review. If there are many credits in each area, 3 or 4 years may be enough. The dean or chairperson should know the institution's system well enough to give competent advice on what will be necessary and how long it will take to accomplish it. Ordinarily, once the number of years until tenure review is agreed upon, it cannot be changed.

Peer Review for Tenure. There is no universally accepted policy for peer review in terms of who conducts or participates in the process and who is evaluated, criteria interpretation, the nature of the process itself, or goals of the process (Porth, 1978). Often, the tenured faculty of a department reviews the evaluation materials, which the nontenured faculty member has submitted and makes initial tenure recommendations to the dean. In the years preceding the final tenure review, this takes the form of a progress-toward-tenure report and recommendations to retain or not retain the faculty member. Utilizing the tenured faculty for this task relieves nontenured faculty from competing with one another for tenured positions or making decisions in which they have vested interest (Porth, 1978). It also relieves the dean from making the decisions alone. In some departments, the tenured faculty also make salary and promotion recommendations. In others, this is done by administration. Once the tenured faculty has made its recommendations regarding a faculty member, the final decision is usually made by administration.

Use of the tenured faculty to evaluate nontenured faculty can cause problems. When tenure was first established in many institutions, everyone on the faculty received tenure just because they were there. Standards have gradually changed, but many of those individuals who were tenured with few or no standards are still in place as tenured faculty members. Therefore, tenured faculty members may not meet the criteria by which they are now evaluating other faculty. Another problem is that the tenured faculty may not be reviewed or evaluated annually. This can cause resentment. Many institutions do have an annual review of tenured faculty, although this may be done by the dean or chairperson only. Power is a major issue in tenure reviews. There is a great deal of power inherent in tenure decisions. The tenured faculty must make every effort to apply the criteria fairly (Brannigan & Burson, 1983).

Specific Considerations Regarding Tenure. The needs of the specific nursing program should weigh heavily in tenure decisions. For example, a department, which has five positions for medical-surgical faculty and does not anticipate any increase in enrollment or faculty would be unwise to tenure five medical-surgical faculty members. This leaves no room for infusing new ideas. The fit of the faculty member to the school is also an important consideration. Perhaps the person is an excellent faculty member, but the fit is just not right in this job. The faculty member should not take that personally, but benefit by suggestions that are given and seek another position until the fit is right. There is no shame in not being tenured. One can move on to another position and eventually find a superb fit.

Inbreeding is another problem in hiring and in tenure. The National League for Nursing (NLN) specifies that there will be diversity in the preparation of faculty in order to promote the dissemination of ideas. Its accreditation criteria states in part that the reviewers determine if the school's "faculty . . . preparation represents varied academic institutions" (National League for Nursing, 1982). Despite this policy, inbreeding continues as a problem. It has been postulated that this may be due to reduced recruitment budgets and to reduced mobility in society in general. Kornguth and Miller (1985) assert, "Inbreeding is unchecked in schools of nursing." Inbreeding definitely affects hiring in nursing departments of universities.

Employability is greatly enhanced if a potential faculty member's degrees are earned from a variety of universities. Attending universities in different geographic locations is also helpful. Even if a person with several degrees from the same local university is hired and does a good job, he or she is unlikely to be tenured.

Financial exigency is another major factor in tenure quotas. Universities are experiencing decreasing enrollments due to a drop in college-age population and lowered federal and state funds, as well as fewer available grants and private sources of funding (Bobbitt, 1985). As a result, they are attempting to avoid tenuring more faculty members than they will need in the next few years. The cost of a nursing program is also a consideration. Nursing education costs more per student than most other programs, due to the necessary low student-faculty ratio. Some schools are considering dropping their nursing programs due to high cost and low enrollment.

Other Privileges

Leaves of absence are granted to faculty members in most institutions. Policies regarding leaves of absence vary. In some institutions, if the faculty member becomes ill or otherwise unable to work during his or her contract, that semester becomes a paid leave of absence upon the dean's recommendation. In other institutions, the faculty member must apply for a leave of absence. Most leaves of absence that are applied for are unpaid leaves of absence. The difference between an unpaid leave of absence and not working for the university is that during an unpaid leave of absence, benefits such as insurance, tenure, and seniority may continue, where they would not if employment were terminated and the person later re-employed. The faculty member should check the institution's faculty handbook or policy book for specific guidelines regarding leaves of absence.

Sabbaticals are often eagerly looked forward to by faculty members. Contrary to some beliefs, however, a sabbatical is not automatically forthcoming after seven years of teaching. A university may grant a sabbatical for one or two semesters when the faculty member has a specific project in mind, such as writing a book or being a guest faculty member at another institution. The faculty member must apply for the sabbatical and declare what his or her project will be during the time away from the institution. At the end of the sabbatical, the results of the project or teaching must be reported. Salary during sabbaticals varies. Some are at full salary, some at half salary or another percentage of the salary, and some are at no salary. Even if there is no salary, the university faculty member retains the same seniority, tenure, and benefit privileges as the person on unpaid leave of absence.

Retirement guidelines vary by institutions. The faculty member must usually have been at the institution a number of years to qualify for retirement benefits. If the faculty member has been there many years, the position of emeritus faculty may be declared at the retirement rank, such as Associate Professor Emeritus. With this status, the faculty may be able to continue some university privileges, such as access to library and recreational facilities of the university. Faculty handbooks and policy books should be consulted regarding specific guidelines for retirement.

REFERENCES

Abruzzese, R. (1984). Continuing education needs of faculty. *Dean's Notes, 5*(3), 1–3.
Allen, G. R. (1979). *The agile administrator.* Tempe, Ariz.: Tempe Publishers.
American Association of Colleges of Nursing. (1986). *Essentials of college and university education: A working document.* Washington, D.C.: American Association of Colleges of Nursing.
American Association of University Professors. (1975, Summer). Statement on teaching evaluation. *AAUP Bulletin,* 200–202.
American Nurses' Association. (1976). *ANA code for nurses.* Kansas City, Mo.: American Nurses' Association.
American Nurses' Association. (1985). *Facts about Nursing, 84–85.* Kansas City, Mo.: American Nurses' Association.
Bauder, L. (1982). Balancing organizational demands with human needs: The ironic emphasis in schools of nursing. *Western Journal of Nursing Research, 4*(2), 153–165.
Bobbitt, K. C. (1985). Systematic faculty evaluation: A growing critical concern. *Journal of Nursing Education, 24*(2), 86–88.
Bolles, R. N. (1981). *The three boxes of life and how to get out of them.* Berkeley, Calif.: Ten Speed Press.
Bolton, E. (1980). A conceptual analysis of the mentor relationship in the career development of women. *Adult Education, 30*(4), 195–207.
Bowen, H. R., & Schuster, J. H. (1985). Outlook for the academic profession. *Research Dialogues, 1,* 1–7.
Brannigan, C. N., & Burson, J. Z. (1983). Revamping the peer review process. *Journal of Nursing Education, 22*(7), 287–289.
Breen, P. (1981). 76 career-related liberal arts skills. *American Association for Higher Education, 34*(2), 9, 16.
Butts, P. A., Berger, B. A., & Brooten, D. A. (1986). Tracking down the right degree for the job. *Nursing and Health Care, 7*(2), 91–95.
Carpenito, L. J., & Duespohl, T. A. (1981). *A guide for effective clinical instruction.* Rockville, Md.: Aspen.
Chamings, P. A. (1984). Ranking the nursing schools. *Nursing Outlook, 32*(5), 238–239.
Chamings, P. A., & Brown, B. J. (1984). The dean as mentor. *Nursing & Health Care, 5*(2), 88–91.
Collins, N. W. (1983). *Professional women and their mentors* (pp. 7–8). Englewood Cliffs, N.J.: Prentice-Hall.
Curran, C. L., Habeeb, M. C., & Sobol, E. G. (1981). Selecting a doctoral program for a career in nursing. *Journal of Nursing Administration, 11,* 35–37.
Darling, L. W. (1986). Self mentoring strategies. *Nurse Educator, 11*(1), 24–25.
Darling, L. W. (1985). Mentor matching. *Nurse Educator, 10*(4), 18–29.
Farabaugh, N. (1984). Do nurse educators promote burnout? *International Nursing Review,* 47–48, 52.
Farmer, C. H. (1976). College evaluation: The silence is deafening. *Liberal Education, 62*(3), 433–436.
Fawcett, J. (1980). Editorial. On development of a scientific community in nursing. *Image, 12*(3), 51–52.
Fortunato, R. T., & Waddell, D. G. (1981). *Personnel administration in higher education.* San Francisco: Jossey-Bass Publishers.

Frain, M., & Valiga, T. (1979). The multiple dimensions of stress. *Topics in Clinical Nursing, 1*(1), 43–52.
Grandjean, B. D., Bonjean, C. M., & Aiken, L. H. (1982). The effect of centralized decision making on work satisfaction among nursing educators. *Research in Nursing and Health, 5,* 29–36.
Greenwood, E. (1957). Attributes of a profession. *Social Work, 3*(II), 45–55.
Hagerty, B. (1986). A second look at mentors. *Nursing Outlook, 34*(1), 16–19.
Hamilton, M. W. (1981). Mentorhood: A key to nursing leadership. *Nursing Leadership, 4,* 4–13.
Herman, J., McArt, E., & Belle, L. (1983). New beginnings: A study of faculty career changers. *Improving College and University Teaching, 31*(2), 53–60.
Hinds, P. S., Burgess, P., Leon, J., McCormick, H. J., & Svetich, L. (1985). Self identified stressors in the role of nursing faculty. *Journal of Nursing Education, 24*(2), 63–68.
Jacox, A. (1976). The community of scholars: Its meaning and the involvement of nurse faculty. In L. Sams, To what extent are nursing faculty a part of the community of scholars in higher education? *Current issues affecting nursing as a part of higher education* (p. 31). New York: National League for Nursing.
Jeglin-Mendez, A. M. (1982). Burnout in nursing education. *Journal of Nursing Education, 21*(4), 29–34.
Kadner, K. (1984). Change: Introducing computer-assisted instruction CAI to a college of nursing faculty. *Journal of Nursing Education, 23*(8), 349–350.
Karuhije, H. F. (1986). Educational preparation for teaching: Perceptions of a nurse educator. *Journal of Nursing Education, 25*(4), 132–144.
Kelly, L. Y. (1985). *Dimensions of professional nursing* (5th ed.) (p. 332). New York: Macmillan.
Koltz, C. J. (1979). *Private practice in nursing* (p. 41). Germantown, Md.: Aspen.
Kornguth, M. L., & Miller, M. H. (1985). Academic inbreeding in nursing: Intentional or inevitable? *Journal of Nursing Education, 24*(1), 21–24.
Krampitz, S. D., & Williams, M. (1983). Organizational climate: A measure of faculty and nurse administrator perception. *Journal of Nursing Education, 22*(5), 200–206.
Lenhart, R. C. (1980). Faculty burnout and some reasons why. *Nursing Outlook, 28*(7), 424–425.
Lenz, E. R., & Waltz, C. F. (1983). Patterns of job search and mobility among nurse educators. *Journal of Nursing Education, 22*(7), 267–273.
Liebler, J. G. (1983). Job descriptions: Development and use. *The Health Care Supervisor, 1*(2), 23–30.
MacPhail, J., & Munro, M. F. (1983). Orientation to academia: The socialization of new faculty. *Nursing Paper, 15*(3), 43–47.
Mauksch, I. G. (1982). The socialization of nurse faculty. *Nurse Educator, 7*(4), 7–10.
May, K. M., Meleis, A. I., & Winstead-Fry, P. (1982). Mentorship for scholarliness: Opportunities and dilemmas. *Nursing Outlook, 30*(1), 22–28.
Megel, M. E. (1985). New faculty in nursing: Socialization and the role of the mentor. *Journal of Nursing Education, 24*(7), 303–306.
Meisenhelder, J. B. (1982). Networking and Nursing. *Image, 14*(3), 77–80.
Mills, W. C. (1983). Orientation to academia: The socialization of new faculty. *Nursing Paper, 15*(3), 21–42.
Moore, L., Damewood, D. M., Floyd, C., & Jewell, K. (1984). A method for achieving quality assurance in nursing education. *Nursing and Health Care, 5*(5), 269–274.

Muldary, T. W. (1983). *Burnout and health professionals: Manifestations and management.* E. Norwalk, Conn.: Appleton-Century-Crofts.

National League for Nursing. (1977). *National League for Nursing criteria for the appraisal of baccalaureate and higher degree programs* (4th ed.). New York: NLN.

Porth, C. (1978). Peer review for nursing faculty. *Journal of New York State Nurses Association, 9*(4), 48–53.

Puetz, B. E. (1983a). *Networking for nurses.* Rockwell, Md.: Aspen.

Puetz. B. E. (1983b, May). Networking hints: Getting organized. (p. 14) *Nurse Educator's Opportunities and Innovations,* Wakefield, Mass.

Ray, G. J. (1984). Burnout: Potential problem for nursing faculty. *Nursing & Health Care, 5*(4), 218–221.

Sams, L. (1976). To what extent are nursing faculty a part of the community of scholars in higher education? In *Current issues affecting nursing as a part of higher education.* New York: NLN.

Schlotfeldt, R. M. (1985). *The N. D. program: Vision for the future.* Cleveland: Case Western Reserve University.

Schriner, J. G., & Harris, I. (1984). Professionalism among nurse educators. *Journal of Nursing Education, 23*(6), 252–258.

Seigel, H. (1986). Expanding the armamentarium for faculty development. *Journal of Nursing Education, 25*(3), 126–128.

Smith, C. E., Baasch, L., & Hoffman, S. E. (1984). Back to the bedside in clinical workshop for nurse educators. *Journal of Continuing Education in Nursing, 15*(2), 45–48.

Smith, M. M. (1982). Career development in nursing: An individual and professional responsibility. *Nursing Outlook, 30*(2), 128–131.

Snyder-Halpern, R. (1984). Doctoral preparation: Is nursing guilty of ethnocentric thinking? *Journal of Nursing Education, 23*(7), 316–317.

Spengler, C. D. (1982). *Networking vital to nursing research.* Paper presented at Fifth Biennial Eastern Conference on Nursing Research, Baltimore, University of Maryland School of Nursing.

Stephenson, C. (1980a). *Sample classroom visitation appraisal.* Dallas: Faculty Affairs Committee, Baylor University School of Nursing.

Stephenson, C. (1980b). *Sample guidelines for faculty self-evaluation reports.* Dallas: Faculty Affairs Committee, Baylor University School of Nursing.

Stephenson, C. (1980c). *Sample opinionnaire regarding academic advisor.* Dallas: Faculty Affairs Committee, Baylor University School of Nursing.

Stephenson, C. (1980d). *Sample opinionnaire regarding classroom instructor.* Dallas: Faculty Affairs Committee, Baylor University School of Nursing.

Stephenson, C. (1980e). *Sample opinionnaire regarding clinical instructor.* Dallas: Faculty Affairs Committee, Baylor University School of Nursing.

Stephenson, C. (1980f). *Sample peer evaluation of committee work.* Dallas: Faculty Affairs Committee, Baylor University School of Nursing.

Sullivan, M. J. (1985). Faculty evaluation: Our shackle or parachute? *Nursing & Health Care, 6*(8), 447–448.

University of Connecticut Personnel Policies. (1978). *Blue Book.* Storrs, Conn.

University of Massachusetts. (1978). *Red book: Academic policies of the University of Massachusetts at Amherst.* Boston and Worcester: University of Massachusetts.

University of Texas, School of Nursing. (1983). *Faculty handbook.* (p. 48) San Antonio: University of Texas.

Urbano, M. T., & Jahns, I. R. (1986). A developmental approach to doctoral education. *Journal of Nursing Education, 25*(2), 76–78.
Vance, C. (1982). The mentor connection. *Journal of Nursing Administration, 12,* 7–13.
Van Ort, S. R. (1985). *Teaching in collegiate schools of nursing.* Boston: Little, Brown.
Veninga, P. L., & Spradley, J. P. (1981). *The work stress connection: How to cope with job burnout.* Boston: Little, Brown.
Wakefield-Fisher, M. (1985). Locus of decision making in schools of nursing. *Journal of Nursing Education, 24*(2), 82–83.
Wakefield-Fisher, M. (1983). The issue: Faculty practice. *Journal of Nursing Education, 22*(5), 207.
Wandelt, M. A., Duffy, M. E., & Pollock, S. E. (1985). *Profile of a top ranked school of nursing.* New York: NLN.
Welch, M. S. (1980). *Networking: The great new way for women to get ahead* (pp. 27, 147). New York: Harcourt, Brace, Jovanovich.

9

Forecasting Future Careers

Margaret Denise Zanecchia, Ph.D., R.N.

Forecasting the future careers for nurse educators in the college or university system is possible through a process called *futuring*. Futuring is a method for determining how probable events might affect individuals (Bell, 1985). The aspects of careers are predictable for nursing educators as individuals or as members of a group of faculty or for nursing education-at-large. Determining the needs of future nurses, students, curriculum, faculty and the issues affecting health care is useful in forecasting trends about the future of nursing education. The identification of newer potential students and the knowledge necessary for a contemporary curriculum of the 1990s is an initial forecasting task (Brimmer, 1984, p. 9; Carty & Bednash, 1985).

FUTURE NURSES

Forecasting the number of nurses needed in the future and the nursing faculty needed is a critical concern. The ratio of employed nurses to the United States population was 356 per 100,000 people in 1970. The number increased to 600 per population in 1983 (American Nurses' Association, 1985). Currently the ratio is 502 per 100,000, i.e., one nurse for 199 people in the United States. (United States Department of Health and Human Services, 1986). The ratio is further projected to increase to 740 per 100,000 in 1990.

However, the health care industry is in crisis. The current problem is the inadequate supply of registered nurses to meet the demand. In 1985, 6.3 percent of the registered nurse positions available in hospitals were vacant. By 1986, that percentage had climbed to 13.6 percent. Both private and public institutions were involved and all the nursing specialties were represented (American Organization of Nurse Executives, 1987).

The gap between supply and demand has increased and a severe shortage exists. Although the shortage of nurses in the early 1980s has curtailed, some nursing leaders are predicting another national nursing crisis beginning in 1987 (Rosenfeld, 1987, p. 283). In 1977, the supply of registered nurses in the United States was 1.4 million and 70 percent were employed full time. (Morrissey, 1987b, p. 358). A supply of 1.7 million actively employed nurses was projected to meet the needs at the end of 1990 (United States Department of Health and Human Services, 1984, pp. 21–23). By 1984 there were 1.9 million registered nurses with more than 79 percent in the workforce. A major shortage of baccalaureate and higher-degreed nurses exists and is anticipated to continue at least until the year 2000.

The Institute of Medicine study (1983) recommends increasing the number of nurses with master's and doctoral degrees in nursing. While nursing has often been envisioned as an occupation of mainly hospital workers, (Blaney, 1986, p. 183), college-bound nurses are needed who are not representative of typical hospital nursing. Nurses with degrees beyond the baccalaureate are needed for many of the innovative positions within occupational health, high-tech clinical care and health care administration (McCarthy, 1986, p. 5). Approximately 358,000 nurses with a graduate education were predicted as needed in 1989 (United States Department of Health and Human Services, 1984), and only 118,000 will have earned this higher degree (McCarthy, 1986, pp. 5, 16).

The United States currently has 360,000 nurses who hold baccalaureate or higher degrees in nursing. With 750,000 of these degreed nurses needed by the year 2000, critical educational needs continue to exist. Actually, the projected need would be far greater than that (Styles & Holzemer, 1986, p. 5). The deficiency projected by the Federal government is 600,000 nurses by the same year (United States Department of Health and Human Services, 1985).

FUTURE STUDENTS

Nursing students of the 1980s are different from those of the earlier decades. Many are older, may have already earned a college degree, and may be men. Some have families, some are already nurses and more minorities are represented (Young, 1985, p. 227). The nursing students of the future may be very different from yesterday's and today's students. Future students will probably represent more diverse backgrounds, broader economic ranges and various countries of origin. They will probably be bilingual and computer literate (Goodman & Alexander, 1984).

Future students will continue to be older adult learners, married or single parents, or single. They may have a previous degree though not in nursing. A market continues to exist for the non-nurse college graduate. Eight college-graduate nursing programs are established for college graduates who are not yet registered nurses but who seek a master of science in nursing as the first professional degree. Of a total 131,017 admissions, 5500 were applications from previously degreed college graduates. Advanced degrees, 90 master's and 12 doctorate, were held by those enrolled, according to Slavinsky et al. (1983). Future students of nursing are certain to be as challenging for faculty to teach as those students of the past.

The 18-year-old female cohort is shrinking due to population shifts. Also, other more attractive and higher-salaried career positions are selected by the contemporary high school graduate. Because of these trends, the potential number of students enrolling in nursing programs is reduced. Nevertheless, in 1982–1983, an increase of 4.8 percent existed in admissions to initial registered nurse programs. (National League for Nursing, 1983; NLN, 1984; ANA, 1985, p. 122).

The student admissions to the three types of basic nursing programs in 1982–1983 included:

- Diploma 19,368, or 15.8 percent
- Associate degree 64,831, or 52.9 percent
- Baccalaureate and higher degree 38,334, or 31.3 percent

Approximately 8 percent of female high school graduates chose nursing as a career in that same year, representing an increase from 6.9 percent in the prior years (ANA, 1985, p. 116). With the numbers of basic students increasing in nursing, there was a gain in the number of programs over those existing in 1982. However, the 1490 basic programs are forecasted to decrease in number during the 1990s and some have already been closed. The applicant number has been reduced by 26 percent since 1984 and the number of graduates is projected to drop 15 percent by 1990 (Morrissey, 1987a, p. 198).

Enrollments in 1983 totaled 254,723 students, a gain of 3.8 percent over the previous year (ANA, 1985, p. 117). In 1983, the number of nursing candidates who took the National Council Licensure Examination for Registered Nurses (NCLEX-RN) for the first time was 83,133. In 1985, annual admissions to basic nursing programs fell 4.5 percent from 1984, down to 118,200. Diploma programs dropped approximately 17 percent from the previous year. Associate degree programs declined 4.2 percent and baccalaureate programs maintained an increase of less than 1 percent. The enrollments fell 8 percent from 1984 and 13 percent from 1983. The losses for diploma programs were 19 percent; associate degree, 8 percent; and baccalaureate 4 percent over the previous year. Fall admissions for 1986 reveal an 8.8 percent decrease to about 83,000, the lowest fall admissions since the year 1970 (Morrissey, 1987b, p. 283).

The total number of graduates is projected to drop. (Mallison, 1985). The total graduations were projected as follows:

- 1990: 18,000
- 1995: 60,000
- 2000: 58,000

Baccalaureate Students

Some 76 percent of nurses who are employed may return to school on a part-time basis seeking a baccalaureate or higher degree in nursing. Also, the more than 286,568 nurses not employed and not now seeking employment may become a future college market. At the same rate of employment, approximately 75 percent or 1.2 million nurses could return to school for a higher nursing degree creating an increased market.

Forecasting probable new baccalaureate-student markets is also predictable from the admissions data for the associate and diploma nursing programs. In 1981–1982, the number of students entering nursing programs was 245,509 (ANA, 1985, p. 136). Since approximately two thirds of these students do not enter the baccalaureate program, they can be considered in long range planning and as a future potential market for the baccalaureate degree. In 1983, 151,612 students enrolled in basic programs other than the baccalaureate (NLN, 1984, p. 30). In the United States in 1984, the number of baccalaureate programs accredited by the National League for Nursing was 352 or 81.3 percent (ANA, 1985, p. 118). Baccalaureate graduations of registered nurse students were 9105 in 1982–1983 (NLN, 1984). However, according to a survey by the American Association of Colleges of Nursing (AACN), generic programs graduated 20,703 with 6,189 being R.N.s, to total 26,892 (Redman & Pillar, 1986a, p. 70). The estimated number of employed registered nurses with the baccalaureate degree as the highest educational preparation is 347,100 as of 1983. Nurses with associate degrees and diplomas number 977,180, a potential market for the B.S. degree in nursing (ANA, 1985, p. 20).

Graduate Students

Among the 1,662,382 nurse population in the national R.N. sample are 5 percent who have a master's or doctoral degree (United States Department of Health and Human Services, 1982, p. 2). Potentially all nurses graduating from baccalaureate programs are at some time future markets for the graduate degree in nursing. However, in 1982–1983, the number of nurses awarded the master's degree was estimated to be 5085 (ANA, 1985, p. 118). For the years 1980 through 1983, 35 to 37 percent of the registered nurses earning an academic degree were awarded master's degrees.

The number of graduate programs in the United States is 154, and there are two master's programs in Puerto Rico. Enrollments in master's programs was 18,112 in 1983, an increase of 6 percent (ANA, 1985, p. 118). The majority of enrolled students (over 71 percent) specified advanced clinical practice as the nursing focus. The functional purpose of the program for 13.5 percent was specified as teaching. In 1983, 834 graduated from a master's degree program, with teaching identified as the functional area. Over 3500 specified clinical practice.

A future trend exists for more educational preparation aimed at the higher degree. Formal and informal graduate study is anticipated. The graduate degree will be the requirement for nursing management and administration in all settings.

According to the AACN data (Redman & Pillar, 1986a), 5315 students graduated in 1984–1985. At a rate of 5000 a year, another 30,000 nurses would be prepared to meet the needs projected for 124,200 master's-prepared nurses. Of the actively employed nurses in the year 2000, 214,300 are projected to need master's or doctoral degrees (United States Department of Health and Human Services, 1984, p. c-12).

Graduate nursing programs of the future will more than challenge the student. Successful students will be better able to meet the demands placed on the nursing profession, the largest group of future health care providers. The predictors of their success may guide future admissions of students (Sime, Corcoran, & Libera, 1983; Foxall, Morgan, & Brage, 1984).

Doctoral Students

In 1980, there were approximately 0.2 percent of the nursing population who held the doctorate. Of the estimated 1.7 million R.N. population, only 3400 nurses made up this 0.2 percent (Young, 1985, p. 223).

Of the total number of those graduating with the master's degree, a small percentage becomes the market for a doctoral degree, and a smaller percentage of those select professional nursing education as a career. In 1982–1983, 139 were granted the doctoral degree (NLN, 1984), and in 1984–1985, 203 earned the doctoral degree (Redman & Pillar, 1986a, p. 7).

Enrollments in doctoral programs in 1983–1984 were 1519 (ANA, 1985, p. 119). In the United States, there are 33 doctoral programs (Redman & Pillar, 1986a, p. 9). Approximately 1 percent of the degreed nurses who graduated in 1983 earned a doctorate, up from 0.9 percent in the previous 2 years (ANA, 1985, p. 152). At present, there are approximately 3648 registered nurses holding the doctoral degree (ANA, 1984).

Approximately 5000 doctorally prepared nurses are projected to be needed by 1990. Even though the estimated number of active nurses with master's or doctoral degrees will almost double, there will continue to be a shortfall.

Whether sufficient numbers of graduate students will choose nursing education as a career to meet future demands is unknown. Whether nursing education is projected as an attractive and rewarding career choice for prospective nurse educator remains untold. Will today's nurse educator be prepared to meet the needs of a changing population of entering student nurses at the college level? The newer teaching–learning theories and the care technologies will require all types of innovative teaching expertise if undergraduate and graduate students of nursing are to be prepared to give optimal comprehensive professional care to clients in the coming decades.

FUTURE FACULTY

Because of the "higher-degree" needs in the nursing profession, more nurse educators and more faculty careers are anticipated. Future faculty who are committed to the process of educating students for roles in the leadership of the health professionals are in critical need (Gorr, 1983. p. 484). One of the major commitments of faculty is to the reforming of the health care delivery system into a wellness versus illness system. Nurse faculty are leaders who can provide insight for the necessary educational preparation of these future care givers.

Of the 1.7 million employed nurses in 1980, it was estimated that 3.7 percent or 62,900 faculty were employed in nursing education (Young, 1985, p. 223). The AACN data from the Fall 1985 represented 128,000 students in 367 baccalaureate and graduate programs and their respective faculties (Redman & Pillar, 1986a, p. 1).

Educational Requirements for Faculty

In a survey, it was found that the educational requirement for nursing faculty positions is the Master of Science degree for a limited number of positions. The doctorate is required for 36 percent of the positions and preferred for 58 percent on graduate faculties. From 67 to 71 percent of the positions in educational administration (dean, associate dean, chair, or head) require the doctoral degree (Butts, Berger, & Brooten, 1986).

Although no doctorates were required for faculty in 1972, there is change anticipated. In fact, all faculty may be required to have or to earn the doctoral degree in the next decades. Some faculty, however few, do pursue postdoctorate study during sabbaticals and leaves.

Type of Degree. The type of doctoral degree is becoming more important. While approximately 75 percent of the degrees are Ed.D.s or Ph.D.s in education or educational administration, the current trend is towards the nursing doctorate. The N.D. (nursing doctorate), the D.N.Sc. (Doctorate in Nursing Science), and the Ph.D. (doctor of philosophy in nursing) are expected to increase (Table 9–1).

TABLE 9–1. REGISTERED NURSES WITH DOCTORAL DEGREE: TYPE AND PERCENT (N = 3648)

Degree	Percent
Ph.D.	53.9
Ed.D.	32.5
D.N.S., D.N. or D.N.Sc.	7.0
D.Ph., Dr.Ph., Psy.D.	3.4
J.D.	2.9
Other[a]	0.3

[a]Doctors of medicine, dentistry, osteopathy, and chiropractic (*American Nurses' Association*, 1985, pp. 11–12).
From American Nurses' Association Center for Research, Statistics and Data Analysis (1984). A special calculation from data collected for the 1984 directory of nurses with doctoral degrees.

Age of Faculty

Nurses with doctoral degrees number 3648. Those with doctoral degrees range in age from below 30 years to above 60 years. The mean age range is 45–49 years; however, another 19 percent are between 40 and 44 years (ANA, 1985, p. 80). Those 50 years and above number 1442, or about half of the supply. Replacement predictions of the older groups due to attrition should create a new demand for doctorally prepared senior faculty.

Salaries for Faculty

The supply–demand of nurse educators may be influenced by the number of faculty with the terminal degree. Faculty salaries increase with higher degrees and higher ranks (Table 9–2). For several years, the report on salaries of faculty and deans has been compiled by the American Association of Colleges of Nursing (1986, p. 11).

Other salary information is compiled by the American Association of University Professors (AAUP), which categorizes institutions of higher learning for data analysis. Depending on the category of the university, the salary is correlated. Several graduate nursing programs are often found in Category I type institutions.

The definition of a Category I university is given by the AAUP.

> These are institutions characterized by a significant level and breadth of activity in and commitment to a doctoral-level education as measured by the number of doctorate recipients and the diversity in doctoral-level program offerings. Included in this category are those institutions that are not considered specialized schools and which grant a minimum of thirty doctoral-level degrees. These degrees must be granted in three or more doctoral-level programs (American Association of University Professors, 1985).

Salaries vary in different regions of the country, with different types of colleges and programs, and with the number of students. The salaries in Category I universities, for example, could be higher than in a college. Salaries may be higher for faculty teaching graduate students and when more students are enrolled in the programs. Usually, faculty salaries are contracted for nine months, an academic year.

TABLE 9–2. AVERAGE FACULTY SALARY BY RANK AND DOCTORATE

Faculty	Doctorate ($)	Without Doctorate ($)
Professor	40,239	37,597
Associate Professor	32,840	30,872
Assistant Professor	28,350	26,273
Instructor	24,116	22,692

Adapted from American Association of Colleges of Nursing, 1986.

TABLE 9–3. AVERAGE SALARIES OF NURSING DEANS BY DOCTORAL DEGREE

Degree	Average Salary ($)
D.N.S. or D.N.Sc.	47,000
Ed.D.	49,300
Ph.D.	52,700
D.Ph. or Dr.Ph.	47,100
Other doctorate	49,700
Nursing Master's	43,100
Other Master's	39,400

Adapted from American Association of Colleges of Nursing, 1986.

The salaries of nursing deans by doctoral degree are shown in Table 9–3.

In 1984, the salaries of deans ranged from under $30,000 to over 70,000 (Young, 1985, p. 333). Salaries of deans, too, vary by tenure, rank, number of programs, numbers of students, and type of university. Of the 383 member schools reporting dean salaries in Fall 1985, the highest annual salary for the dean was $72,800 (Redman & Pillar, 1986b). Salaries are usually based on the calendar year, in contrast to the usual faculty salary based on the academic year.

For college educators, a moderate increase was noted in the last few years. The future salaries are expected to increase only slightly. In the 1970s and 1980s, the salaries in the academic profession have declined by about 16.5 percent, whereas other occupational groups on the average have gained about 3 percent (Bowen & Schuster, 1985, p. 2).

Future Outlook for Faculty

Professional nursing, a traditionally female occupation with the largest number of health care employees, has developed into a career choice with significant future economic and employment opportunities. Future demand and the positive occupational outlook for nurses influence an emerging new role for the nurse educator.

With so many careers open to women, nursing education may not be as enticing as it has been in the past. Yet a competitive demand continues to exist for the number of faculty positions available for professional nurse educators. If the declines in general population materialize, enrollments in nursing could change. The profession may face a continuing critical national shortage of nurses and nursing faculty through the year 2000 and beyond.

Nursing student enrollments in higher education are declining, although admissions to doctoral programs in nursing have increased over the years. Increasing needs for nursing leaders may mean more need for nurses and nursing programs. However, there is always a demand for high-quality, well-prepared faculty to teach the student of the future regardless of the number of students in nursing programs.

The need prevails for more faculty in order to correct faculty turnover and retention rates in addition to the increasing numbers of faculty retirements. Comprehensive recruiting plans, which encourage potential nurse educators to complete higher-degree education, will increase the applicant pool. The demand for nurse educators will likely continue to increase despite the escalating cost of higher-degree programs.

FUTURE CURRICULUM

Futurists have been interested in a quality curriculum, which spans the new century, and in a balancing of a technological and humanistic preparation for health professionals. High demands for new knowledge and skills have produced a knowledge explosion. Little opportunity exists for orderly, thorough, or consistent curriculum development. (Fitzpatrick, 1987, p. 213; Heaney 1987, p. 219).

Nurse educators are needed with the educational preparation for teaching in master's and doctoral programs, autonomous practice, and teaching sophisticated management and administrative skills to students. These needs have implications for change and new emphasis in nursing curricula.

Trends in the development of present graduate curricula have continued and emphasized the functional areas of theory-based advanced clinical practice. Graduate curricula offer the administration of nursing service or educational administration as a focus. Doctorally prepared nurses are needed in nursing service and nursing practice. If the nursing programs met the demands for qualified nurse administrators, an additional 3400 graduates from doctoral-degree programs would be needed (Fine, 1983). At the present rate of over 200 per year, it could take 12 more years to meet this need.

Curricula Levels

The thrust for two levels of nursing, professional and technical, has implications for future nursing educational programs and curriculum. The baccalaureate degree is necessary for professional nursing pursuits, while the associate degree would establish an associate nurse. Potential markets for the B.S. degree exist in the group of A.D. nurses.

The many technical nurses prepared as licensed vocational nurses may also become a potential future market. A curriculum plan to integrate these nurses into the higher education system is sought in some states (Poteet & Hodges, 1986).

Extended Roles

Curriculum implications emerge with the newer extended wellness role and the critical care roles of the nurse. Within nursing practice, nurses have functioned at many levels and in a variety of roles. These roles include maintaining quality of consumer advocacy, research, and more recently, risk management.

The increase of health care in the community dictates the acute care needs in the curriculum. Sicker clients are discharged earlier to homes. Families face a critically ill relative often without the support of nurses.

Wellness and health promotion are also major contemporary roles for the nurse. Nursing curriculum address prevention and holistic care. Demands for a higher level of health and for a higher quality of life exist. Courses explore the risk factors of life-style and prevention as affect morbidity and mortality.

Interdisciplinary Curriculum

Nurses function interdependently in a collaborative manner with others. Nurse leaders interact with many health care professionals through collaboration, including the medical and administrative groups. A major recommendation made by the National Commission to Study Nursing and Education was the formation of a National Joint Practice Commission. The purpose of the group was to provide a forum for nurses and physicians to further collaborate on improving client care. The interaction of the nursing and medical professions has a positive effect even in the face of the physician glut. Predictions are that more than 700,000 physicians will be practicing in the United States by the year 2000, a 54 percent increase from 1980. This rapid growth will produce a surplus of between 20,000 and 70,000 physicians by 1990 (Andreoli & Musser, 1985, p. 47).

Jointly implemented curricula that paired nursing and medical students have enhanced care. Interdisciplinary socialized student teams that have been used effectively in the community setting could be implemented in other settings. The result of educating nursing and medical students together is a greater understanding of the differences of the two groups (Turnbull, 1981, p. 42).

How well physicians and nurses interact may have future implications for clients' lives. A study of 5000 clients in 13 hospitals found decreased rates of death in intensive care units with increased communication and interaction between nurses and physicians (American Nurses' Association, 1986). The limitations of physicians may create more opportunities for nursing (Roncoli & Whitney, 1986, p. 531).

Educational Settings

The total community at large is considered an educational setting for the nursing students of the future. The appropriate learning laboratory settings are wherever the future clients are found.

The elderly comprise 11 percent of the United States population. The increasing aged population is at home or hospitalized in an acute care unit or long-term care setting (Duyeno, Stark, & Kliewer, 1985). Teaching gerontologic nursing was an identified objective for nursing education in the Institute of Medicine report (1983, pp. 171–172).

Well, older clients provide challenging opportunities for teaching preventive health maintenance. These clients are served in wellness centers and other types of faculty-managed programs or clinics housed in the university community (Hawkins, Igou, et al., 1984).

When students learn to care for clients in dyads with faculty, the professional socialization is facilitated. Homebound hospice clients were such a group serving as clinical learning laboratory (Eakes & Burnette, 1986). Day surgery, health fairs, birthing centers, preschool day care, student health centers, outreach programs, shelters for the homeless, and senior centers are used as nontraditional settings for nursing students.

The young and adult well population is in the school or occupational setting. Although more than 70 million Americans engage in some form of self-care activities, the school and occupational nurses are not yet able to be reimbursed for providing health promotion activities (Andreoli & Musser, 1985; Lancaster, 1986). This may change with the legislation for third party payment.

Approximately 100 nurse-managed centers exist, and most are located in schools of nursing (Lang, 1983). Whether they will survive in the future is uncertain. Often the funding source is grant-related. Research and evaluation is necessary to demonstrate the worth of these centers not only as an economical care-giving approach, but as a viable learning laboratory for future nursing students (Barger, 1985). However, the American Medical Association opposes the community nursing centers.

Nursing homes have been and will continue to be a setting for the learning experiences of nursing students. There are 15,000 nursing homes in the United States, and an estimated 30 billion dollars is spent annually. Nursing homes and retirement centers can also serve as settings for teaching students to teach clients wellness and health promotion.

The nation has more than 6000 home health agencies. The home care industry is proliferating. Although visiting nurses, school nurses, occupational health nurses, and public health nurses have served collegiate education in the past, more are expected in the future. As home care grows, more nurses are needed who can teach technological care in the home setting. The home care nurse of the future is a skilled critical care nurse with a background of experience in community health nursing. The future evaluation of home health personnel against standards is mandated (National League for Nursing, 1986), and will ensure quality of care.

Of the 123 academic health centers in the United States, most will remain future settings in the next decade. Seventy-five sponsor a nursing program (56 public and 19 private). Because of greater research activities and larger volumes of clients, the university medical centers will continue to be a viable setting for future nursing students. However, increased funding for health care and tighter federal budgets may influence some (Ebert & Brown, 1983; Schmidt, 1983). Nursing students and other allied health professionals will compete for scarce learning experiences.

Sufficient clinical agencies for placement of nursing students is a current concern and will continue to be a dilemma (Hawkins, 1985). Coordination and innovative scheduling will relieve some congestion, but future nursing students may rotate shifts for client learning opportunities as they once rotated shifts to give client care.

Consumers as clients are demanding and may refuse "to have students" as care givers. Regionalization compounds the problem of specialized care for the client. Future nursing students may be assessed fees for clinical laboratories, a new cost factor for nursing education. However, the transfer of these fees to the clinical agency will offset the cost of time for nursing staff. Nursing service is assessing the inherent loss of supporting a nursing program.

Curriculum Innovations

Graduate curricula focus on specialization and have for several years. However, the idea of a postbaccalaureate degree as the first professional degree in nursing is challenging to curriculum experts. Students graduating from baccalaureate programs would continue and be enrolled in a master's program. While the past B.S. degree would have prepared a nurse as a beginning professional, now the M.S.N. is the first professional degree (Conway-Welch, 1986).

Specialization has been the purpose of graduate education, but a newer curriculum model to prepare the master's degree nurse as an advanced generalist is proposed. Specialization had meant breadth and depth of knowledge in a special problem in the practice field. Lately, a need for an advanced level of generalized knowledge and practice has emerged.

Two master's curricula exist: advanced generalist and specialist; M.S.N. advanced generalist and M.S.N. specialist. The advanced generalist engages in comprehensive, holistic nursing and uses diffused roles, skills, and strategies (Reed & Hoffman, 1986).

Challenging the nurse educator of the future is the new nontraditional curriculum offered by the alternative universities. Alternative universities are businesses, industries, government, and the military. These newer degree-granting institutions are attempting to meet social trends and needs of contemporary students (Arlton & Kalikow, 1986). Faculty teaching curriculum in the corporate classroom may affect the future of the profession of nursing. While rank, tenure, and governance are not emphasized, quality instruction and research in the learning process and novel methods of instruction are important.

FUTURE ISSUES AS FORCES

In a survey by the author, the future forces with potential to affect nursing education were ranked. A questionnaire was sent to nurse educators from member schools of the American Association of Colleges of Nursing. Fifty-six percent of the respondents returned 248 usable questionnaires (Zanecchia, 1985). Forces were described as persons, policies, or situations, which could exert power and pressure to influence future nursing education.

Certain major forces were composed of subforces, i.e. resources contained the subforces of number of existing faculty positions, facilities, number of programs, support services and availability of teaching materials. The Health Care Delivery System included subforces of government regulation:

- New delivery models
- Third-party pay for nursing

The supply–demand ratio included subforces of:

- Registered nurse positions
- Nursing student potential
- Nurse educator positions

Society as a major force included the subforces of:

- Cost of health care
- Image of nursing
- Consumerism
- Changing values

Demographically, the sample consisted of 153 nurse educators from the public sector (61.7 percent) and 95 from private programs (37.9 percent). The number of full-time and part-time faculty by level of program included:

Program Level	Full-time	Part-time
Baccalaureate	23.5	6.7
Master's degree	7.9	8.5
Doctoral degree	10.5	23.0

A dean or director position was held by 93 respondents (37.5 percent).

Position	Number	Percent
Dean or director	93	37.5
Assistant dean	11	4.4
Program or level coordinator	34	13.7
Faculty	104	41.9

Assistant professor was the rank held by most responding to the survey:

Position	Number	Percent
Instructor	16	6.5
Assistant professor	89	35.9
Associate professor	73	29.4
Professor	62	25.0
Other	8	3.2

Although most held the M.S.N. degree, 45.6 percent had a doctoral degree:

Degree	Percent
Ph.D. (other)	19.4
Ph.D. (nursing)	7.3
D.N.Sc.	1.2

Degree	Percent
Ed.D.	17.7
M.S. (nursing)	48.4
M.S. (other)	4.0
B.S. (nursing)	0.4
B.S. (other)	1.6

The average number of years of teaching experience was 13.9 years, with the range of 1 to 21 years. Most had been in the present position 3.31 years.

Years	Number	Percent
0–2	26	10.5
2–3	61	24.6
5–6	53	21.4
7–9	49	19.8
10–13	29	11.7
14+	28	11.3

Tenure status of respondents included tenured, 119 (48 percent); tenure-track nontenured, 98 (40 percent); and nontenure-track, 31 (12 percent).

Major forces affecting nursing education included budget, resources, concept of nursing as a profession, administrative control, and the health care delivery system. Social forces, which had less potential to affect nursing education, included changing values, cost of health care, consumerism, the image of nursing, accrediting bodies, and the supply-and-demand ratio (Table 9–4).

Budget and resources ranked highest of the forces with potential to offset nursing education. Major issues facing nursing educators and nursing education are many of the same issues that influence the practice of professional nursing. Future policy decisions in nursing are predictable from the analysis of the labor market and the clinical role of the nurse (Kalisch, Kalisch, & Belcher, 1985). These same policy issues will influence nursing education and are based in education itself, society and the health care system.

Higher Education

Issues affecting nursing education stem from the situation in higher education itself. Higher-education issues for nursing are challenged by two levels of nursing practice. The implementation of alternative nursing programs within the college setting for the transitional nursing student is an important need. Moving up the educational degree ladder challenges the nontraditional baccalaureate students, but the faculty even more, to create the necessary curriculum. Baccalaureate and graduate programs in nursing are fed by these students and the groups are expected to increase in the future.

Nursing education needs to teach a practice based on its theory and clinical nursing research. Research in nursing education is also necessary to learn better

TABLE 9–4. RANKING AND MEANS OF NINE MAJOR FORCES WITH POTENTIAL TO AFFECT NURSING EDUCATION[a]

Ranking	Force	Mean
1.	Budget	2.89
2.	Resources	3.99
	Faculty positions	1.46
	Facilities and support	2.01
	Teaching materials	2.83
3.	Concept of nursing as a profession	4.06
4.	Administrative control	4.22
5.	Health care delivery system	4.99
	Government regulation	1.96
	New delivery models	2.04
	Nursing third-party pay	2.32
6.	Accrediting licensing bodies	5.27
7.	Supply-and-demand ratio	5.45
	R.N. positions	1.75
	Student potential	2.19
	Nurse educator positions	2.36
8.	Society	5.59
	Cost health care	2.19
	Image of nursing	2.32
	Consumerism	2.92
	Changing values	2.95
9.	Size of professional nursing group	7.17

[a]From most to least important.

strategies for teaching and learning and curriculum development (de Tornyay, 1984; Diekelmann, 1986).

Nursing educators are needed who are competent with computers and who can use computers to teach basic and continuing education. Instruction by computer is ranked as a high priority for the nurse educator, both now and in the future (Armstrong, 1986). Future leaders in nursing education should not be handicapped by the computer age and computer use within the education system. Using information and knowledge is a key element in nursing's response to societal needs.

Technology is a priority for nurse educators because of the advancements in knowledge about technical care and information processing needs. Nurse educators must be aware of and accept future developments (McCormick, 1983; Nelson & Carlstrom, 1985).

In keeping with the constant supply of college-educated nurses exiting the system, academia is forced to respond to the consumer of the graduate, the employer. How well the college nursing product meets the demands of society and the expectation of the employer dictates the future needs for graduates.

Societal Issues

Society and the needs of the employer dictate much about the future of nursing education. Current employers advertise for "experienced" nurses. The employers of baccalaureate graduates may require specialists in acute care for the hospital and community setting. Such specialties are expected to emerge, i.e., nurses prepared to give pre- and postoperative care in laser surgicenters (O'Leary, 1986).

Society has generated a growing group of elderly clients and will demand nurses who are knowledgeable care givers. Because there are 28 million Americans aged 65 and older, the elderly constitute approximately 12 percent of the total United States population of 237 million people. By 2030, Americans aged 65 and older should make up 20 percent of the total U.S. population with those 75 and older representing the majority (Andreoli & Musser, 1985).

More emphasis on learning about the care of the elderly, practice based on research, and wellness programs are needed. Nursing educators are needed. Only 25 of 140 graduate programs and 40 of 299 nurse practitioner programs prepare students in geriatric nursing (Shannon, 1985, p. 48).

Health Care System

Health care system issues are influencing nursing education and the role of the nurse educator. These issues include: the client of the future, health manpower, the economics of health care, and the changing health care system, and in addition the issues of who lives, who dies, and who pays.

Future Clients as Health Care Consumers. Clients in the future will be older citizens. The changing health care system is dictating who will pay for the care of older clients. Hospitals and regulations control the movement of a client through the health care system from admission to discharge.

There are demands for nurses who are experts in maternal and child health, especially the high-risk maternity client and the neonate. In 1983, the birth rate was 15.5 per 1000 live births, and the death rate was 8.6. A total of 3,614,000 babies were born (ANA, 1985).

Health Care Delivery. In 1983, the number of hospitals in the United States was 6888, and the number of beds was 1,350,361. Admissions of 38,886,681 accounted for an average daily census of 1,027,716 and 76.1 percent of occupied beds (American Hospital Association, *Hospital Statistics 1984,* quoted in ANA, 1985, pp. 214–265).

Hospitals will decrease in numbers, compete with community hospitals, divide geographically, and more will become long-term care centers. Admissions will fall faster than length of stays.

Nursing homes will continue as a part of the health care system in the year 2000. The senior population will live to be 75 years of age and older. How the elderly can maintain wellness will indicate life-style patterns of living. Retirement centers, nursing homes, and homes in the community will need support from geriatric nurses for health promotion and prevention.

A movement towards promoting wellness at the worksite is escalating. There are more wellness programs expected in existence by 1990. Employers are also concerned with drug testing in the workplace, and the military has instituted mandatory HIV (AIDS) testing.

Health Manpower. The National Center for Health Statistics estimated that 457,500 physicians were in the United States in 1980, 19.7 per 10,000 population. The National Center for Health Statistics projected that by 2000 there will be 704,700, an increase of more than 54 percent over the 1980 estimate (ANA, 1985, p. 260).

The American Medical Association has proclaimed a physician glut and an oversupply of doctors in all specialties. With the evidence that nurse midwives and practitioners provide high-quality care that is holistic and health-promoting and less expensive, consumers may turn even more to the nurses, regardless of the ready doctor supply. The physician glut has implications for future health care delivery and nursing education. Many policy makers believe nurses and other health care manpower may be able to teach self-care and preventive care to clients (Gunn, 1986). However, physicians may attempt to reclaim nursing's turf because of the competition.

Nursing will need to stand firm or lose the opportunities to offer care financed by third-party payers. The National Commission on Nursing Implementation Project is providing a plan that may enable nursing education to remain a part of the new health care system and to anticipate patient needs in that future system (Peck, 1986).

Nursing education must prepare hospital-based nurses to take the leadership role in planning follow-through care at home or long-term care. Community nurses, occupational health nurses and school nurses must be prepared to develop and collaborate on health care programs, which reduce health risk, change life-style, and facilitate wellness for clients (Fagin, 1986).

Economics of Health Care. An estimated 10.8 percent ($355.4 billion) of the 1983 gross national product was spent on health. Health care per capita basis was $1459 in 1983. These data are expected to increase to 12 percent before the year 2000 (ANA, 1985, p. 262).

Hospital systems are changing and will be shaped in the next decade by those who will be the payers. Carol McCarthy (Petitte & Anderson, 1986, pp. 53–54), the president of the American Hospital Association, stated:

> A shift will occur from cost-based reimbursement to a price-driven financing arrangement—the focus on maintaining the delicate balance between cost, quality, and access.

During the 1990s, hospitals are predicted to become computer centers that will link up doctors with their patients for a service charge. Only 10 percent of hospital utilization will be from health maintenance organizations. Most will come from managed premium negotiated rate insurance plans (Petitte & Anderson, 1986). However, approximately 35 million persons in the United States will be uninsured or underinsured.

Consumer groups are now looking at quality and cost for care. The American Association of Retired Persons (AARP) has recognized that substituting nurse-provided care whenever possible is cost-saving. The Association also is interested in a review of the physician payment system (Ostrander, 1986).

SUMMARY

Analysis of societal issues and forces acting on nursing education is an endless task. Future students, future curriculum, and future faculty are important factors. A continuing need exists to define the tasks and responsibilities of *faculty* in nursing education within the context of *service* to society. A balance is sought among the state of the art, the demands of society and the necessary career role forecasted for the nursing educator of the future.

REFERENCES

American Association of Colleges of Nursing. (1986). *Report on nursing faculty salaries 1985–1986* (p. 11). Washington, D.C.: Institutional Data System, American Association of Colleges of Nursing.

American Association of University Professors. (1985). The annual report on the economic status of the profession. *Academe*.

American Nurses' Association. (1984). *1984 directory of nurses*. Kansas City. Mo.: Center for Research, Statistics and Data Analysis.

American Nurses' Association. (1985). *Facts about nursing 84–85*. Kansas City, Mo.: American Nurses' Association.

American Nurses' Association. (1986). ICU patient's life depends on how well RNs, MDs get along. *The American Nurse, 18*(8), 1, 16.

American Organization of Nurse Executives. (1987). *Preliminary report of the 1986 hospital nursing supply survey*. Chicago: AONE.

Andreoli, K. G., & Musser, L. A. (1985). Trends that may affect nursing's future. *Nursing & Health Care, 6*(1), 47–51.

Arlton, D. M., & Kalikow, T. J. (1986). The single purpose road. *Nursing & Health Care, 7*, 36–40.

Armstrong, M. L. (1986). *Present and future competencies for nurse educators in basic and continuing education*. Summary report of dissertation. East Texas State University School of Education.

Barger, S. E. (1985). Evaluating a nurse-managed center. *Nurse Educator, 10*(4).

Bell, D. F. (1985). Futuring: Planning for tomorrow's learner. *Nurse Educator, 10*(3), 4.

Blaney, D. R. (1986). An historical review of positions in baccalaureate education in nursing as basic preparation for professional nursing practice 1960–1984. *Journal of Nursing Education, 25*(5), 182–185.

Bowen, H. R., & Schuster, J. H. (1985). Outlook for the academic profession. *Research Dialogue, 6,* 1–7.

Brimmer, P. (1984). *The economics & employment environment: Recent developments and future opportunities* (p. 9). Kansas City, Mo.: American Nurses' Association.

Butts, P. A., Berger, B. A., & Brooten, D. A. (1986). Tracking down the right degree for the job. *Nursing & Health Care, 7*(2), 91–95.

Carty, R., & Bednash, G. (1985). Tomorrow's nurses. *Nursing & Health Care, 6*(9), 492–496.

Conway-Welch, C. (1986). School sets sights on bold innovations. *Nursing & Health Care, 1,* 21–25.

de Tornyay, R. (1984). Research on the teaching-learning process in nursing education. In H. H. Werley & J. J. Fitzpatrick (Eds.), *Annual review of nursing research* (pp. 193–209). New York: Springer Publishing Company.

Diekelmann, N. L. (1986). Why research in nursing education. *Nurse Educator, 11*(1), 4–5.

Duyeno, L., Stark, A., & Kliewer, E. (1985, October). Forecasting demand for long-term care. *Health Services Research.*

Eakes, G. C., & Burnette, B. (1986). Home-bound hospice as a learning environment for mental health nursing students—a model approach. *Journal of Nursing Education, 25*(5), 217–218.

Ebert, R. H., & Brown, S. S. (1983, May 19). Academic health centers. *The New England Journal of Medicine,* 1200–1208.

Fagin, C. M. (1986). Opening the door on nursing's cost advantage. *Nursing & Health Care, 7*(7), 353–357.

Fine, R. B. (1983). The supply and demand of nursing administrators. *Nursing & Health Care, 10*(1), 10–14.

Fitzpatrick, M. L. (1987). Dimensions of quality in nursing education. *Nursing & Health Care, 8*(4), 213–216.

Foxall, M. J., Morgan, N., & Brage, D. (1984). Challenging graduate nursing students to think for the future. *Journal of Advanced Nursing, 9*(3), 291–295.

Goodman, L. R., & Alexander, M. K. (1984). RN's as nontraditional students: A faculty perspective. *Imprint, 31*(2), 57–63.

Gorr, A. (1983). Introduction: Educating tomorrow's health professionals. In C. McGuire, R. Foley, A. Gorr, & R. Richards (Eds.), *Handbook of health professions education* (pp. 483–485). San Francisco: Jossey-Bass Publishers.

Gunn, I. P. (1986). Nursing innovations help reach traditional goals. *Nursing & Health Care, 7*(7), 359–362.

Hawkins, J. W. (1985). Locating and selecting clinical agencies. *Nurse Educator, 10,* 20–25.

Hawkins, J. W., Igou, J. F., et al., (1984). A nursing center for ambulatory well, older adults. *Nursing & Health Care, 4,* 209–212.

Heaney, R. P. (1987). Standards of quality: The path to excellence. *Nursing & Health Care, 8*(4), 219–221.

Institute of Medicine. (1983). *Nursing and nursing education: Public policies and private actions* (pp. 3, 171–172). Washington, D.C.: National Academy Press.

Kalisch, B. J., Kalisch, P. A., & Belcher, B. (1985). Forecasting for nursing policy: A news-based image approach. *Nursing Research, 34*(1), 44–48.

Lancaster, J. (1986). 1986 and beyond: Nursing's future. *Nursing & Health Care, 16*(3), 31–37.

Lang, N. (1983). Nurse managed centers: Will they thrive? *American Journal of Nursing 83, 9,* 1290–1293.

Mallison, M. B. (1985, February). Editorial. Present imperfect, future tense. *American Journal of Nursing,* 121.

McCarthy, C. (1986, February). Nursing is on the road to health. *The American Nurse, 5,* 16.

McCormick, K. A. (1983). Preparing nurses for the technological future. *Nursing & Health Care, 4*(7), 379–382.

Moccia, P. (1987). The nature of the nursing shortage: Will crisis become structure? *Nursing & Health Care, 8*(6), 321–322.

Morrissey, K. L. (1987a). The nursing crunch is on. *Nursing & Health Care, 8*(3), 198.

Morrissey, K. L. (1987b). The critical case for continued funding of nursing programs. *Nursing & Health Care, 8*(6), 358–359.

National League for Nursing. (1983). *State approved schools of nursing—RN, 1983.* New York: National League for Nursing.

National League for Nursing. (1984). *Nursing student census with policy implications, 1984.* New York: National League for Nursing.

National League for Nursing. (1986). The quest for quality. *Public Policy Bulletin, IV,* 2.

Nelson, J. P., & Carlstrom, J. A. (1985). A new confrontation: Nursing education and computer technology. *Image: The Journal of Nursing Scholarship, 17*(3), 86–87.

O'Leary, J. (1986). What employers will expect from tomorrow's nurses. *Nursing & Health Care,* 207–209.

Ostrander, V. R. (1986). Consumers look to nurses for affordable quality care. *Nursing & Health Care, 7*(7), 369–370.

Peck, S. B. (1986). Nursing on the cutting edge of opportunity. *Nursing & Health Care,* 365–367.

Petitte, K., & Anderson, H. J. (1986). Major systems shaped by payers. *Modern Health Care, 16*(17), 53–54.

Poteet, G. W., & Hodges, L. C. (1986). Guest editorial. Displaced persons in nursing. *Nurse Educator, 11*(4), 5.

Redman, B. K., & Pillar, B. (1986a). *Report on nursing enrollments and graduations in colleges and university.* Washington, D.C.: American Association of Colleges of Nursing.

Redman, B. K., & Pillar, B. (1986b). *Report on salaries of nursing deans 1985–1986.* Washington, D.C.: American Association of Colleges of Nursing.

Reed, S. B., & Hoffman, S. E. (1986). Master's education. *Nursing & Health Care, 7*(1), 43–48.

Roncoli, M. & Whitney, F. (1986). The limits of medicine spell opportunities for nursing. *Nursing & Health Care, 7*(10), 531–534.

Rosenfeld, P. (1987). Nursing education in crisis—A look at recruitment and retention. *Nursing & Health Care, 8*(5), 283–286.

Schmidt, A. M. (1983). Challenges to academic health centers. *Handbook of Health Profession Education.* San Francisco: Jossey-Bass Publishers.

Shannon, K. (1985). Geriatric training lags behind projected demand for employees. *Hospitals,* 48.

Sime, A. M., Corcoran, S. A., & Libera, M. B. (1983). Predicting success in graduate education. *Journal of Nursing Education, 1,* 7–11.

Slavinsky, A., Diers, D., & Dixon, J. (1983). College graduates: The hidden nursing population. *Nursing & Health Care, 4*(7), 378–378.

Styles, M., & Holzemer, W. (1986, February). As I see it, let's remap to avoid educating too many, too few. *The American Nurse,* 5.

Turnbull, E. (1981). Health care issues as an interdisciplinary course. *Nursing Outlook, 29*(1).

United States Department of Health and Human Services. (1984). *Report to the President and Congress on the status of health personnel in the United States.* Washington, D.C.

United States Department of Health and Human Services. (1985). *Fifth Report to Congress.* Government Printing Office.

United States Department of Health and Human Services. (1986). *Fifth Report to the President and Congress on the status of health personnel in the United States: March 1986.* Springfield, VA.

Young, L. K. (1985). *Dimensions of professional nursing* (5th ed.) (p. 223). New York: Macmillan.

Zanecchia, M. D. (1985). Faculty workload elements and forces affecting nursing education. *Proceedings and Abstracts* (p. 34). Third Annual Meeting, Society for Research in Nursing Education, San Francisco.

Index

A

Academic
- advising of students, 21–23, 95–97, 99–100, 106
- freedom, 11, 61, 142–143, 147
- profession, 1–2. *See also* Profession
- ranks, 59, 98, 152, 156–160, 195–197, 203
- roles, 1–2, 6–7, 9–10, 15–34, 41, 54, 57, 59, 69–71, 84–85, 112, 117, 152–161

Accreditation, program, 10, 20, 31, 135

Administration. *See also* Faculty; Nurse-managed health centers
- doctorally prepared, 98, 117, 198
- employment negotiations, 141–142
- position descriptions, 129, 152–155
- faculty relationships, 59, 60, 73, 81, 84, 89, 141, 143, 145, 153–155, 157, 160, 169
- research, 98
- salary, 198
- as service, 20–21, 29–30, 90–91, 102, 154, 155, 159, 160
- workload, 64–67, 87, 91, 98–99, 143, 153–155

Advertisements, classified, 66, 118–119

Advising
- of faculty, 44, 143, 144, 147, 168–170
- career entry, 112
- students. *See also* Advocacy; Counseling
- as service, 95–97
- characteristics, 21–23, 97
- evaluation reports, 181
- faculty mobility, 21, 96
- part-time faculty, 106
- workload, 8, 95–97, 99, 100, 152, 155, 159

Advocacy. *See also* Advising
- patient, 27, 199
- student, 27

Age of faculty, 115, 121, 194–195, 197

Age of students, 192–195

Agencies
- coordination, 28, 145, 155
- faculty relationships, 59, 68, 69, 73, 76–77, 157, 178

American Nurses' Association Code for Nurses, 150

Assessment. *See* Evaluation

B

Baccalaureate degree programs, 26, 86, 90, 120, 144, 192, 194
Baccalaureate nurses, 24, 134, 192–194
Benefits, fringe, 117, 127, 129, 138–139, 140–141, 147, 185
Burnout, 60, 146, 147, 162, 170–172

C

Career. *See also* Profession
  academic, 7, 15–17
  advising, 44, 112, 143, 144, 147, 168–170
  changes, 9, 41–42, 111–112, 117, 118, 146, 162. *See also* Faculty: mobility
  choice, 4, 15, 59, 112, 118, 147
  definition, 112, 149
  development, 8, 9, 32, 69–70, 84–85, 93, 99, 113, 145, 161–166
    definition, 112, 162
  education, 112, 114–115, 117, 125, 164–166
  entry, 6–9, 111–129, 134, 135, 145, 156
  evaluation, 114–115, 118, 144, 146–147
  experience, 134, 135, 145, 156
  goals, 6, 9, 11, 32, 42, 114–115, 116, 144, 172–185
  planning, 42, 112–113, 144, 161–172
  settings, 117–120, 160–161, 200–202
    evaluation, 15, 114–115, 118, 144, 146–147
  strategies, 113–116, 144, 166–172
  values, 116, 146–147
Certification, professional, 114, 122, 125, 145, 146, 162–163, 179
  as professional development, 25, 32, 42, 94–95, 162–163
Characteristics of nurse educators, 1–2, 4–5, 12, 15–34, 40–41, 48, 112–116, 152–153, 160–161, 195–199, 203
  career entry, 42, 113–116
  employment references, 121–122, 144
  workload, 85, 99, 161–162

Classified advertisements, 66, 118–119
Clinical
  evaluation reports, 53–54, 145–146, 178, 179
  expertise, 24–26, 31–32, 62, 93–95, 135, 145–146, 150, 159, 162–163
    loss, 145, 147
    risk reduction, 146–147
    workload, 94, 99, 103
  learning, 2, 18, 27–28, 51–53, 58, 68
  placement of students, 28, 52, 155, 200–202
  practice. *See* Faculty; Nursing practice
  teaching, 2, 19, 51–52, 58, 68, 82, 86–87, 155, 157, 178, 179, 200–202
  workload, 82, 94–95, 103–105
Codes of ethics, 150
Collaboration, 57–78, 88, 150. *See also* Faculty: practice
  agency coordination, 28, 145, 155
  as service, 20–21
  clinical expertise, 145
  workload reduction, 107
Collective bargaining, 142
College
  faculty. *See* Faculty
  functions, service, 26–27, 29–30, 41, 91–92, 156
  reputation, 26–27, 118, 160
  system, model, 3–11
Committees. *See also* Organizations
  as continuing education, 164
  as service, 20–21, 24, 54–55, 83, 127
  faculty, 6, 8, 29–30, 40, 54, 68, 90–93, 142–143, 147, 152–153, 156, 158
  faculty search, 128–129
  local service, 20–21
  workload, 87, 91, 98, 152–153, 156, 158
Communication skills for career entry, 6–9
Communication during interviews, 127–129
Communication in teaching, 41, 68
Community
  organizations, 20–21, 91, 92

service, 7, 9, 20–21, 29–30, 54–55, 62, 64–67, 85, 91–93, 150, 158, 179. *See also* Faculty: practice
  in employment interviews, 127
  levels, 91
  requirements, 158
Competencies, continued, 24–26, 31–32, 93–95, 145, 146, 150, 159
Computer skills, 5, 21–22, 90, 112, 114, 115, 140, 164, 205
Conducting nursing research, 73–76
Conferences. *See also* Organizations: professionals
  career entry, 112
  as service, 31, 88, 90–91, 147
  student clinical, 52–53
  workload, 94
Consulting, 20, 33, 57, 63, 71–72, 76–77, 84, 92, 123, 149
  requirements, 158, 159
  workload, 99
Continuing education, 32, 112, 126, 147, 164–166
Contracts, employment, 129, 136, 138–139, 141–142, 151
Coordinators
  course, 152, 153
  division, 152, 154–155
  level, 152, 153–154
Counseling, 22, 43, 84, 95, 97, 147, 168. *See also* Advising
Course coordinators, 152, 153
Courses. *See* Curriculum
Cover letters, 122–125
Cultural benefits, 141, 147
Curriculum, 8, 23–24, 44–45, 87, 88, 99, 10, 143
  coordinators, 153–154
  evaluation, 23–24, 40, 45
  part-time faculty input, 67–68, 106
  trends, 44–45, 199–200
Curriculum vitae, 125–127
  definition, 125

D

Deans. *See* Administration
Department heads. *See* Administration

Development
  career, 8, 9, 32, 58–59, 69–70, 84–85, 93, 99, 113, 145, 161–166
  definition, 112
  for doctorally prepared faculty, 111, 117, 147
  for non-doctorally prepared faculty, 32, 93, 95, 111
  professional, 31–32, 41–42, 94–95, 112, 113, 147, 161–166
Division coordinator, 152, 154–155
Doctorally prepared faculty, 93, 98, 111, 117, 134, 135, 144, 196, 198. *See also* Nondoctorally prepared faculty
  employment outlook, 117, 119, 162–164, 196, 202
  research, 89
  salary, 198
Doctorate nursing programs
  for faculty, 115, 163–164
  in nursing, 26–27, 50, 86, 90, 111, 115, 120, 194–195
Dress, 115, 127, 156, 157

E

Economic costs
  of education, 20, 26, 51, 62, 81, 96, 101, 141, 143, 145, 147, 163
  of health care, 24, 59, 69, 147, 207–208
Editing, 20, 88
Education. *See also* Teaching; Development
  continuing, 126, 147, 164
    as professional development, 32, 112, 164–166
  continuing education unit (CEU), 32, 126, 165–166
  for career, 112, 114–115, 117, 125, 164–166
  costs, 20, 26, 51, 62, 81, 96, 101, 141, 143, 145, 147, 163
    advising effects, 22, 96
  faculty qualifications, 135, 144, 156, 157, 158, 159, 196
  as professional development, 31–33

216 INDEX

Education (*cont.*)
  programs, 26–27, 50, 86, 90, 111, 115, 120, 144, 163–164, 192, 194–195, 199–202
  requirements, nursing programs, 18
  resources, 58, 68–69, 83, 84–85, 127, 140, 154, 166
  settings, 18, 144, 200–202
  skills, 5, 9, 164–165, 199–200. *See also* Teaching–learning process
  computer, 5, 21–22, 112, 114, 115, 164, 205
  social change, 117, 206
Employment
  acceptance, 40–41, 129
  applications, 122–125
  changes, 111, 117, 118, 146, 160–161
  contact names, 31, 120, 125
  contracts, 129, 136, 138–139, 141–142, 151
  cover letters, 122–125
  curriculum vitae, 125–127
  dress, 115, 127, 156, 157
  experience, career entry, 113–115, 134, 135, 145, 156
  guides, 117
  interviews, 124, 127–129, 140
    role playing, 127
  opportunities, 59, 117, 119, 120, 133, 145, 149, 191, 204–205
  outlooks, 116–117, 191–208
  placement services, 119
  politics, 33, 142–143, 183–184, 206–208
  positions, 11, 15, 118, 127, 137, 153–159
  qualifications, 40, 41, 145, 196
  references, 121–122, 144
  rewards, 138–147, 182, 185
  risks, 60–61, 116, 138–147, 162, 170–172, 182
  search, 116–129
    records, 125
    strategies, 121
  search committees, 128–129
  settings, 15, 40, 140, 160–161, 200–202
  telephone canvases, 119, 123, 124
  tenure, 129, 182. *See also* Tenure

  thank-you notes, 129
  transcripts, 122
Environmental forces. *See* Forces in nursing education; Roles
Ethics, codes, 150
Ethics, teaching of, 47–48
Evaluation
  career, 114–115, 118, 144, 146–147
  of curricula, 23–24, 40, 45
  employment interview, 127–129
  of faculty, 154, 172–182
    clinicals, 53–54, 145–146, 178, 179
    criteria, 173–174
    data included, 174–179
    methods, 9–10, 172–173, 174–182
    outcomes, 174
  of practice, 60, 63, 69, 71, 95
  reports, 40
    administrative, 178
    agency, 178
    peer, 176–179
    self, 174–175
    student, 146, 178, 179
  of research, 19–20, 88, 183
  of service, 21, 23, 91–92
  of teaching, 40, 175–178, 179, 180
  tenure requirements, 70, 136–137, 143–144, 182–183, 184
  using workload formulas, 54–102
  part-time faculty, 106, 138, 142
  peer review, 176–179, 183–184
  of pending positions, 11, 15, 118, 127, 133
  of students, 26, 28, 50–54, 72, 146, 154, 157, 158
Experience
  for career entry, 113–115, 134, 135, 145, 156
  in career change, 113–115
  positions, 153, 155, 157, 158, 159

F

Faculty
  adjunct, 59
  advising. *See* Advising
  age, 115, 121, 194–195, 197

assignments, 59, 69–70, 97, 100–101, 103, 142, 152. *See also* Committees
burnout, 60, 146, 147, 162, 170–172
characteristics, 9–10, 12, 15–34, 40–41, 112–116, 152–153, 160–161, 195–198, 203
doctorally prepared, 89, 93, 98, 111, 117, 119, 134, 135, 144, 147, 162–164, 196, 198, 203
educational requirements, 135, 144, 156, 157, 158, 159, 196
employment risks and rewards, 133–147
evaluation. *See* Evaluation
manual, 141, 151
mix, 106–107
mobility, 112, 117–118, 146. *See also* Employment changes
effect on advisees, 21, 97
nondoctorally prepared
employment opportunities, 117, 119
preparation, workload, 93, 111, 136–137, 140–141
professional development, 32, 93, 95, 111
release time, 141–142
tenure risks, 137, 144–145
part-time, 59, 106, 138, 142, 145, 147, 182, 202–203
peer review, 176–179, 183–184
practice, 57–78, 145, 165
characteristics, 9, 24–29, 49
evaluation, 60, 63, 69, 71, 95
as professional development, 25, 94
role model, 62–63
workload, 94–95, 99, 158
productivity, 9–10, 81–107, 140–141
professional development, 31–32, 41–42, 94–95, 112, 113, 147, 161–166
qualifications, 144, 146, 150, 153, 154, 155, 156, 157, 158, 195–196
ranks, 59, 98, 152
characteristics, 156–160, 195–197, 203
recruitment, 61, 103, 120
relationships

administration, 59, 69, 73, 81, 84, 87, 89, 141, 143, 144, 145, 153–155, 157, 160, 169
agencies, 59, 68, 69, 73, 76–77, 157, 158
college, 9–10, 26, 40–41, 72, 81, 84, 141, 142, 145, 155, 156, 158
peer, 20, 41, 63, 68, 71, 82, 89, 142–143, 147, 150, 167–168, 183–184. *See also* Mentors
physician, 92, 112
student, 6, 12, 18, 21–22, 49, 52, 60, 71, 96, 128, 145–146, 150, 155
roles, 1–2, 6–7, 9–10, 15–34, 41, 54, 57, 59, 69–71, 84–85, 112, 117, 152, 161
search committees, 128–129
socialization, 16, 89, 90, 191
subsystem, 6–7, 9–10
tenure, 32, 69–72, 136–140, 144–145, 182–185
Fellowships as professional development, 93
Forces in nursing education, 10–12, 20–21, 33, 81, 82–83, 111, 117, 134, 145
Formulas, workload, 100–102, 105
Fringe benefits, 117, 127, 129, 138–139, 140, 141, 147, 185
Future in nursing education, 12, 117, 134, 144–145, 191–208. *See also* Career

G

Goals, 16, 69, 93, 147. *See also* Motivation
advising, 21–23, 96
career entry, 42, 114–115, 116, 144–145, 160–166, 172–185
of educational systems, 9–10, 40, 154, 185
learning, 32
Governing councils, 29–30, 142–143, 147, 152
collective bargaining, 142
Graduate degree programs, 25–27, 58,

Graduate degree programs (*cont.*)
  86, 102, 111, 115, 120, 134, 136, 144, 192, 194–195, 199
Graduate students, in faculty workload reduction, 106, 140
Grants, 9, 118, 162
  as professional development, 88, 93
  in workload formulas, 87, 102
  writing, 19, 88
Grievances, 142, 146
Guidance, student, 22, 41, 83, 97, 146. *See also* Advising

H

Handbooks, manuals, guides. *See* Career; Education; Faculty
Health care. *See also* Nursing care
  as service, 20–21, 92, 158
  costs, 24, 59, 69, 147, 207
  delivery, 147, 200–202, 206–207
Health centers, nurse-managed, 64–67, 92, 200–207
Health needs in society, 201–202, 206
History of nursing education, 39
Human resources
  in colleges, 10, 140, 151
  mentoring, 34, 43–44, 168, 170

I

Instruction. *See* Teaching
Insurance
  fringe benefits, 138
  professional, 138, 145–146
Interacting System Model, 1–13, 15, 23, 82, 101
  and career entry, 113, 114, 115
Interpersonal relationships. *See* Faculty; Relationships
Interviews, employment, 124, 127–129, 140

J

Job. *See* Employment
Joint appointments, 59–78. *See also* Collaboration
  for clinical expertise, 25, 145
  and licensure, professional development, 94
  workload, 92

L

Lecture anxiety, 48
Lecture methods, 46–51
  discussions, 48–50
Level coordinator, 152, 153–154
Licensure, 9, 51, 94
  examination writing, 134–135
Litigation
  faculty, 138, 142, 145–146, 147
  student, 145–146
Local community service, 20–21, 91–93, 145. *See also* Service

M

Marketing, 26–27
  employment position, 117–118, 120–121
Master's-prepared faculty, 32, 93, 95, 111, 117, 119, 136–137, 140–142, 144–145
Meetings. *See* Committees
Mentoring, 34, 43–44, 168–170. *See also* Preceptorships
Methodology, teaching, 44–54
Merit, 72, 83, 137–138, 139, 147. *See also* Evaluation
Models, 2–12, 61–65, 71, 76, 85. *See also* Interacting System Model; Systems
Mobility, faculty, 21, 97, 112, 117–118, 146
Morale, faculty, 6, 141, 143, 146, 147, 162, 170–172
Motivation, 40, 41, 85, 95, 112–113, 118, 133, 147, 161–162. *See also* Goals

N

Negotiating contracts, 129, 136, 138–139, 141–142, 151

Networking, 20, 21, 147, 167–168
  employment search, 118, 120
  references, 121–122
Nondoctorally prepared faculty, 32, 93, 95, 111, 117, 119, 136–137, 140–145
Noninstructional responsibility, 15–17, 54, 57–78, 84–85, 88–97, 99, 149–172
Nonverbal communication, interviews, 127–128
Nurse-managed health centers, 21, 64–67, 92, 200–201
Nurse–physician relationships, 200
Nursing care, 68, 71, 199–202, 206–208. *See also* Health Care
  needs, 114, 191–192, 206–208
  quality, 68–69, 145
  standards, 67–68, 71
  trends, 146, 205, 206–208
Nursing faculty. *See* Faculty
Nursing practice, 7, 10–12, 24–26, 59–62, 68, 71, 73–74. *See also* Faculty: practice; Teaching
  as service, 21, 147, 158
Nursing programs, 26–27, 39, 50, 55, 86, 90, 111, 115, 120, 134, 155, 163–164, 191–208

O

Office space as benefits, 140
Organizations. *See also* Committees; Governing councils; Unions
  community, 20–21, 91, 92
  faculty, 90–91, 142, 147
  frameworks, research, 68–74
  professional, 6, 10, 17, 30, 31, 91–92, 150. *See also* Committees
    in employment searches, 120
    information about, 154
    presentations, 19, 103
    service, 54, 84, 91–92
    tenure aspects, 143
    workload, 99, 100, 104–105
  presentations, 19
  student. *See* Student support services

Orientation, faculty, 7, 40–41, 43–44, 143, 153, 154, 168, 151
Orientation, student, 151, 155, 157. *See also* Advising

P

Part-time faculty, 59, 106, 138, 142, 145, 147, 182, 202–203
Patient education, preparation for career entry, 114
Peer review, 176–179, 183–184
Personal
  characteristics, 4–5, 16, 33, 40–41, 48, 113–114, 115, 116. *See also* Profession characteristics
  needs, 115, 133, 192–193
  references, employment, 121
  satisfaction, 12, 17, 25, 42, 55, 58, 147, 160–161
Personnel, 10, 140
  bulletins, employment, 119–120, 138
  contacts, employment, 31, 120, 125, 138–139
Philosophy
  educational, 15–16
  in interviews, 127
  nursing, 15–16, 23, 134
  of teaching, 40, 42–43
Physician–nurse relationship, 200
Physician–nurse educator relationship, 92, 112
Placement services, 119
Planning, career, 42, 112–113, 144, 161–172
Policy. *See also* Politics; Organizations; Governing councils; Health care
  college manual, 40, 141–142, 185
  coordinators, 154–155
  of educational programs, 61, 140
  faculty, 40, 106–107, 151, 185
  grievances, 146
Politics, 12, 33–34, 87, 142–143, 160, 183–184, 206–208
  college settings, 29–30, 142, 146
Position descriptions, 151–160
Practice. *See* Faculty: practice; Nursing practice

Preceptorships, 27–28, 44, 106. *See also* Mentoring
Presentations, 19, 128–129
  as service, 103, 156
  as professional development, 94
Prestige
  of colleges, 118, 161
  as faculty, 2, 141, 142, 147
Probationary periods, 138–139, 141, 144, 183
Productivity, 9–10, 81–107, 140–141. *See also* Evaluation; Promotion
  strategies, 105–107
Profession
  academic, 1–2
  characteristics, 1–2, 4–7, 15–17, 40–41, 81–82, 84–85, 99, 112–113, 150, 160–161, 195–199
  of practice, 24–26, 94–95
  certification, 25, 32, 42, 114, 122, 125, 145, 146, 162–163
  definition, 1–2, 112, 150
  development, 31–32, 41–42, 93–95, 111–113, 147, 161–166
    as faculty practice, 95, 146
    certification, 25, 42, 94–95, 162–163
    requirements, 7, 158, 164–165
    workload, 94–95, 99
  employment references, 121–122, 144
  liability, 138, 145–146, 147
  organizations. *See* Organizations
  roles. *See* Roles
Promotion, 72, 83, 99, 142. *See also* Evaluation: of faculty; Tenure
  collective bargaining, 142
  service aspects, 69
  steps, 137–138, 139
Publishing, 9, 12, 19, 25, 55, 83, 85, 88, 98–99, 146, 183. *See also* Promotion
  and doctorally prepared faculty, 89
  requirements, 41, 143, 158, 159, 183
  tenure aspects, 20, 143, 146, 183

Q

Qualifications. *See* Career; Faculty

R

Rank, faculty, 59, 98, 152, 156–160, 195–197, 203
Reappointment, collective bargaining, 142
Recommendations, employment, 121–122, 144
Records in employment searches, 125
Records for evaluation, 40, 172–182
Recruitment of faculty, 61, 103, 120
Recruitment of students, 26–27, 55, 199
References, employment, 121–122, 144
Referrals, employment, 31, 119–120
Relationships. *See also* Faculty; Students
  nurse–physician, 200
  physician–nurse educator, 92, 112
Release time, 89, 140–142, 185
Reports, as service, 55, 92. *See also* Evaluation
Reputations, colleges, 26–27, 118, 160
Research, 7, 9, 12, 18–20, 41, 57–78
  career entry, 112, 117, 118–120, 133
  computers, 90, 112, 115, 140
  conducting and utilizing, 73–76
  of doctorally prepared faculty, 98
  effect on advising, 96
  evaluation, 19–20, 88, 183
  quality enhancement, 55
  resources, 74, 89, 140
  space as a benefit, 140
  in teaching, 19, 72
  for tenure, 144, 183
  workload, 83, 84, 88–90, 99–105, 158, 159, 160, 161
Responsibilities, 11–12, 15–34, 41, 66–67, 70, 83–85, 99, 144. *See also* Roles
  of part-time faculty, 106
  of position descriptions, 153–160
Resumes, 125–127
  definition, 125
Retirement
  fringe benefits, 138, 140, 147
  guides, 185
Rewards of employment, 23, 31, 40, 55, 58–60, 116, 138–147, 182, 185. *See also* Personal: satisfaction; Salary

Risks
  of advocacy, 27
  of employment, 60–61, 116, 137–147, 162, 170–171, 182
  reduction, 146–147
Roles. *See also* Politics; Service in society, 58–59, 91–92, 133, 147
  academic, 1–2, 6–7, 9–10, 15–34, 41, 54, 57, 59, 69–71, 84–85, 112, 117, 152–161
  role modeling, 25, 33, 44, 60, 63, 71–72, 92, 151, 168
  role playing for interviews, 127

S

Sabbaticals, 140, 185
Salary, 135–136, 147. *See also* Rewards
  annual raises, 136, 137–138, 139, 142
  employment interview, 127, 129
  information sources, 117, 136
  negotiations, 69, 70, 72, 77
  part-time faculty, 59, 106
  steps, 137–138, 139
  trends, 197–198
  workload formula, 100–101
Satisfaction. *See* Personal; Career
Scholar, definition, 150–151
Scholarly activities, 2, 18–20, 32, 41, 62, 69, 71, 88–89, 144, 150–151. *See also* Research
  workload, 83, 98–99, 102–103
Scientific community, 150
Search committees, employment, 128–129
Seminars
  as professional development, 94, 112
  as service, 31, 92
Service, 16–17, 54–55, 84. *See also* Roles; Faculty
  administrative, 20–21, 29–30, 90–91, 102, 154, 155, 159, 160
  community, 7, 9, 20–21, 29–31, 54–55, 62, 64–67, 85, 90–93, 147, 150, 158, 179
  college, 7–8, 26–27, 29–30, 41, 54, 62, 90–93, 142–143, 156, 158, 159, 160

definition, 20–21, 54, 90
as development, 94
employment interviews, 127
evaluation, 21, 23, 88, 183
levels, 91
position requirements, 158
professional, 54, 58, 62, 99, 161
seminars, 31, 92
student advising, 95–97
tenure aspects, 144
time requirements, 39, 55, 104–105, 158
Sexism in academia, 30, 98, 161–162
Skills
  for career entry, 6–9, 41, 113–116
  computers, 5, 21–22, 90, 112, 114, 115, 140, 192, 205
  educational, 5, 9, 164–165, 199–200
  maintenance as professional development, 93–94, 145
Social
  benefits, 55, 129, 141, 147, 206
  needs, 11–12, 23, 45, 111, 117, 191–192
  systems, 6–7, 10–11, 133
Socialization, 16, 89, 90, 151
Society, 10, 23–24, 206–206. *See also* Roles
Standards. *See* Promotion; Politics
Student
  advising, 21–23, 95–97, 100, 151, 152, 155, 159
  age, 192–193
  baccalaureate, 192–194
  characteristics, 50–51, 192–195
  clinical placements, 28, 52, 155, 200–202
  doctoral, 194–195
  evaluation, 26, 28, 50–54, 72, 146, 154, 157, 158
  faculty relationships. *See also* Advising; Role models
    elements of, 6, 12, 18, 21–22, 49, 52, 60, 71, 96, 128, 150, 155
    litigation, 54, 145–146
    workload, 36, 99–100, 156, 157, 158
  outcomes of faculty productivity, 101, 174

Student (cont.)
  progress, 8–9, 50–51, 53–54, 156–157
  student–student relationships, 49
  support services, 7–8, 91
Supervision, 6, 82, 87–88, 157. *See also* Teaching
  employment references, 121–122
  of students, to maintain clinical expertise, 26, 95
Surveys
  American Association of Colleges of Nursing, 59, 99
  faculty workload, 32, 99
  forces in nursing education, 119, 202–203
  teacher characteristics, 41
Systems. *See also* Models
  curriculum, 8–9
  faculty, 6–7, 9–10
  individual nurse educator, 4–5, 113–116
  model, 2–11
  student, 7–8
  theory, 11

T

Tasks. *See* Workload
Teachers. *See* Faculty
Teaching, 39–55, 81, 83. *See also* Roles; Teaching–learning process
  assignments, 69–70, 101–102, 142
  assistants in workload reduction, 106
  characteristics, 18, 40–41, 85–88
  clinical, 2, 19, 51–52, 58, 68, 82, 86–88, 155, 157, 178, 179, 200–202
  college, 87, 111
  conditions, 84–85, 147. *See also* Governing councils; Working hours; Workloads
  definition, 87–88
  evaluation, 40, 175–178, 179, 180
  expectations, 40, 42, 156
    faculty, 41–43
    institutional, 40–41
  experience qualifications, 114, 136, 144, 156–159
  history, 39
  position requirements, 144, 152, 156–159
  quality enhancement, 9, 24, 58–59, 67–68, 90, 164–166
  team, 45, 81, 153
  tenure aspects, 144
  workload predictor, 82, 100–105, 142
Teaching–learning process, 7, 16, 23–24, 27, 42, 60–61, 63. *See also* Roles; Teaching
  for career entry, 114, 128
  quality enhancement, 22, 41, 66
Team teaching, 45, 81, 153
Telephone
  canvassing for employment opportunities, 119, 123, 124
  references for employment, 122
Tenure, 32, 83, 93, 99, 147, 182–185. *See also* Promotion
  clinical aspects, 26, 69–70, 72, 144
  collective bargaining, 142
  credit toward, 137, 182
  definition, 136, 182
  employment interviews, 129
  evaluation, 40, 175–180, 182–184
  expectations, 136–137, 139–140, 144–145
  faculty mix, 107
  not obtaining, 144, 182, 184–185
  risks, 137, 144–145, 182
  service aspects, 30, 144
Test anxiety, 50–51
Testing, 50–51
Thank you notes
  in evaluation, 179
  for interviews, 129
Theory
  development, 19
  learning, 42–43
  lecture methods, 46–47
Transcripts, 122
Transitions. *See* Forces in nursing education; Careers
Tuition, fringe benefits, 138, 147
Tutoring, 28–29. *See also* Advising; Teaching

U

Unions, 10, 142

V

Values, career selection, 116, 146–147, 150

W

Working hours, 84, 85–86, 100–106, 133. *See also* Teaching
Workloads, 25, 51, 55, 81–107. *See also* Surveys; Teaching
  analysis, 98–100
  clinical, 82, 94–95, 99, 103–105, 107, 146–147, 158
  doctoral preparation, 93, 111, 136–137, 140–141, 144
  employment interviews, 127, 142
  formulas, 100–102, 105
  position description, 152–153
  self-reporting, 98
  strategies, 105–107, 170–172
  student advising, 8, 95–97, 100, 152, 155, 159
  survey, 32, 99
  time, 5, 87–88, 93, 97, 99, 102, 103–104, 105, 137, 152
Workshops
  career entry, 112
  as professional development, 94, 147–179
  as service, 31, 55, 92, 179